COLOR WAR

DINSHAH P. GHADIALI'S BATTLE WITH THE
MEDICAL ESTABLISHMENT OVER HIS
REVOLUTIONARY LIGHT-HEALING SCIENCE

STEVEN M. RACHLIN, M.D.
HARVEY RACHLIN

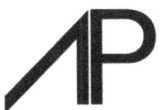

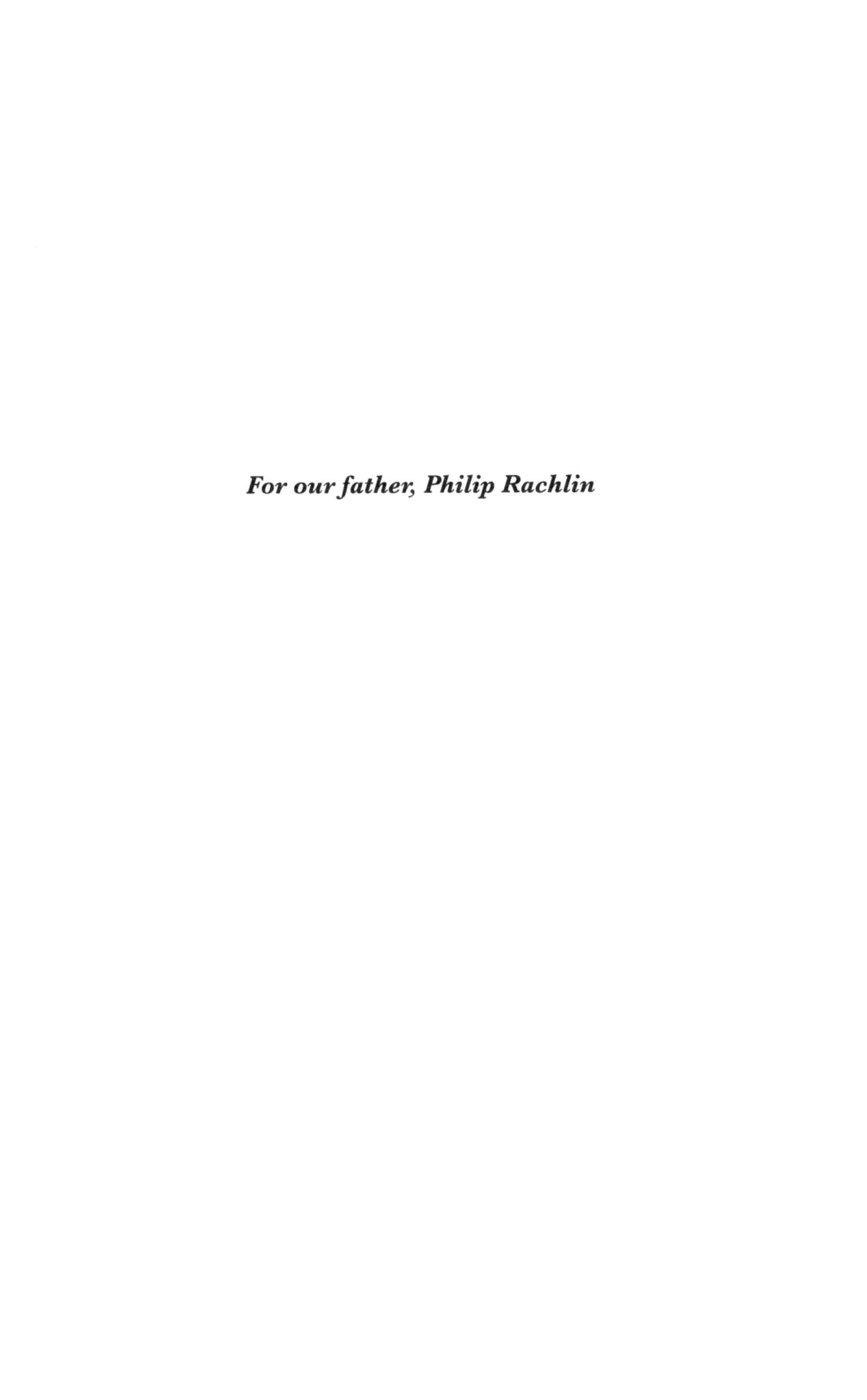

For our father, Philip Rachlin

CONTENTS

INTRODUCTION

Color War: Dinshah P. Ghadiali's Battle with the Medical Establishment over his Revolutionary Light-Healing Science is the story of a man who in 1920 introduced a new healing art. He believed he had perfected a method to cure many human diseases and ailments, and demonstrated his work to physicians, surgeons, dentists and other health professionals who subsequently used it with astonishing results. They reported the successful treatment of cancer, high blood pressure, diabetes, tuberculosis, rheumatism, arthritis, asthma and numerous other diseases. This man claimed the results obtained with his unconventional healing science far surpassed those of orthodox medicine.

As expected, the organized forces of medicine set out to stop him. They tried every which way, repeatedly bringing him to court; he was jailed ten times. Followers of his science also suffered. One prominent physician, the senior surgeon at the oldest women's hospital in America, practiced the science for several years with the full support of the hospital's board. After a disparaging article about this man's healing methods appeared in the *Journal of the American*

Medical Association, the interns at the hospital forced the senior surgeon to resign.

The subject of our story is Dinshah P. Ghadiali, a Parsee Indian who made himself known by his first name (pronounced din' shä) after he found Americans had trouble pronouncing his last name. Dinshah was considered brilliant in his lifetime by both friends and adversaries. His healing science was based on principles of light and color and he called it Spectro-Chrome Therapy. Color therapy was not new, having been practiced in one form or another for centuries. But Dinshah reported that after many years of intensive research he had brought empirical trial-and-error therapy to scientific precision.

Within five years of introducing Spectro-Chrome, Dinshah had trained, by his estimation, some 2,000 health professionals and laypersons in his healing art. Adherents to this science wrote numerous case histories of sufferers treated with it. Dinshah published thousands of these in his monthly journal. Some physicians stated that Spectro-Chrome worked so well that reporting case histories was redundant. Spectro-Chrome received unanimous praise from its myriad users.

For many years Dinshah constantly challenged the American Medical Association to investigate his methods. He stated that if Spectro-Chrome was proven effective he would donate his patents to the U.S. Government for the benefit of mankind; if proven ineffective he would leave the U.S. and never return. The challenge was never accepted. Instead, he was constantly brought to court. In one trial Dinshah was accused of grand larceny and in others he was accused of practicing medicine without a license; many of his trials received national media attention.

The American Medical Association has been one of the most powerful lobbying groups in Washington, spending millions of dollars yearly to protect and improve its members' interests. Thus the monumental if not impossible task Dinshah faced in having Spectro-Chrome Therapy investigated can be readily appreciated since his therapy posed a direct threat to organized medicine and drug companies.

Dinshah devoted years of intensive research to determine that diseased organs have abnormal emanations (auras) and that they can be "normalated" (remedied) by applying appropriate "attuned color waves" (color waves of certain oscillatory frequencies calculated to coincide with those of the cells of the human body). Using spectroscopical techniques, Dinshah was able to determine the chemical imbalance of diseased organs (whether the imbalances were excessive or deficient) and what color wave radiations may neutralize auras of diseased organs and bring them back to a normal state. No drugs or surgery are used in Dinshah's system, only a projector with an incandescent white light and five colored slides, so it is unlikely to induce any adverse side effects. Unlike drugs, which have a systemic effect after digestion, attuned colors would be applied only locally over the diseased organ in many cases.

Color War tells the remarkable life story of Dinshah, his science of Spectro-Chrome Metry, his thoughts on nutrition and metaphysics, and his struggles against the powerful "medical trust." Whether he was right or wrong with his science, Dinshah's journey into the mainstream world of health care with his unconventional form of healing that was fervently followed by legions of physicians all over America is an exciting, controversial and unforgettable story.

Dinshah's Platform - as adopted by him in 1891

The boundless oscillatory ocean of thought is essentially universal and all-pervading; it is the individualized monopoly of no person and is the common heritage of humanity's evolution; thus, what a development of unrevealed ages has given unto me in the form of knowledge in my present incarnation is no distinctive acquisition of mine for my sole use, benefit or elevation, but is all for thee and is thine without condition, without obligation, without expectation. I fear no one; only God above and conscience below and from them I have nothing to fear.

1

A NEW HEALING SCIENCE MAKES ITS DEBUT

Lectures were a popular amusement in 1920, and, on Monday, April 26, the hall in New York City where Dinshah was about to speak was comfortably filled. Many in the audience were curiosity seekers — miraculous cures were always interesting; there might even be some gruesome or salacious slides — but among them were more serious listeners. Some knew Dinshah, who had been a colonel in the New York Police Reserve and Governor of the Police Aviation School. Others knew him as a fellow member of the American Association of Progressive Medicine. Still others knew him by reputation as a brilliant orator and something of a genius.

The mass of the audience was surprised, however, to see a small, dark-skinned man in what looked like pajamas decorated with bright medallions, and with a brilliant purple skullcap on his head, mount the podium. There was an uneasy shifting, even a few titters, which were hushed by embarrassed or better-informed neighbors. They quieted when Dinshah began to speak. It was obvious that English was not his native language because of the charming lilt of his voice, but his speech was perfectly clear and fluent.

It was also convincing to those who listened with open minds.

Dinshah briefly described his many years of research on a new healing process called Spectro-Chrome, beginning with his desperate attempt as a 24-year-old in India to help a young woman afflicted by severe mucous colitis whose case was adjudged hopeless by other physicians. Since the woman had already been treated by all conventional methods without result, Dinshah resolved to try a procedure described by Dr. Edwin Dwight Babbitt, a New York physician, in *Principles of Light and Color*. It seemed mad, perhaps, that shining colored light on a person could cure colitis — but surely it could do no harm, and every other treatment had already failed.

To Dinshah's own amazement, the woman was soon well enough to resume her daily routine. Perhaps, Dinshah admitted, she had been cured by her own hope of a cure — ignorant people often are better treated by what they believe is "magic" than by science — but it was equally possible that the colored lights had had an effect. Dinshah began to experiment, sometimes on cases considered utterly hopeless, like his first attempt, sometimes on conditions that were sufficiently mild that no danger to the patient could develop from lack of other treatment.

There were failures; Dinshah was feeling his way, learning the effects of different colors, of different times of exposure — all the variables of a new procedure of treatment. But there were successes too. And, as his management of the procedure and his rate of success improved, he became so positive of the validity of his therapy that now, Dinshah said triumphantly, he was prepared to offer a perfect healing process — Spectro-Chrome — to the public without clinical testing.

Dinshah then described the science of color waves in detail. It was as exact a science as any medical treatment could be, Dinshah claimed with calm conviction when members of the audience clustered around him after the lecture was over. Dinshah also pointed out that this science could never produce an adverse reaction, although in the reparative process there may be temporary discomfort such as a rash or diarrhea.

Neither the enthusiastic presentation on the lecture podium nor his spirited replies to the questions showered on him by both interested and antagonistic listeners betrayed Dinshah's inner qualms. He had no doubt about his healing process. He was ready to stake his life on its efficacy! In fact, that was just what he was doing — staking his life on Spectro-Chrome. Dinshah was a genius, not a fool. But he knew that if he was successful in convincing a large number of people that Spectro-Chrome could meet his claims he would meet fierce opposition from the forces of organized medicine.

Over the past few years, after he himself had been convinced of the marvels that Spectro-Chrome could produce, a war had raged within his soul. Dinshah knew that if he kept his knowledge to himself he could remain safe, even respected, treat people and probably grow rich. Private treatments would not be challenging orthodox medical practices openly. But private treatments could reach only very, very few people. Even if he did not try to grow rich, even if he ministered to the needy for free, he could reach only a tiny fraction of the sick. Thousands would suffer and die, who, Dinshah was certain, could have been alive and well if treated with Spectro-Chrome.

Fear urged Dinshah to tread the path of caution, to treat those he could, to introduce Spectro-Chrome to those open-minded and sympathetic doctors who would try before condemning. Compassion and, yes, pride, urged Dinshah in the other direction. Caution was not a characteristic of his nature. From the time he had challenged his father by reading "forbidden" Western books and conducting scientific experiments to his emigration to a country prejudiced against those with dark skin he had never been guided by caution. Compassion, on the other hand, had been a driving force all his life — and there was pride also.

To introduce Spectro-Chrome publicly, to claim openly that his process would eventually prove superior to orthodox medical practice was a dangerous gamble. If he succeeded deathless honor would be his. His name would be known along with those of Hippocrates,

Galen, Lister and Pasteur; he would never be forgotten. If he failed, he would be ruined and dishonored. Even so, thousands would have learned about Spectro-Chrome before the forces of organized medicine began to take him seriously and mount their attack on him.

Now one, now the other argument prevailed, but more and more as Spectro-Chrome proved its worth Dinshah came to feel that whatever the cost to himself, he could not withhold so valuable a science of healing from the public. Thus was born the lecture given on April 26, 1920 and others that followed at different locations around New York City.

At first all went well. Not only was each audience sufficiently interested to question Dinshah, but some people even bought his machines. Of these, a few were physicians and surgeons and they — some to their own amazement — reported spectacular results. Others told Dinshah that they were interested in trying Spectro-Chrome but did not trust themselves to follow the instructions or interpret the results correctly. They felt they needed more instruction than could be furnished in a single lecture.

Dinshah was delighted with this idea. It was true that Spectro-Chrome could do no harm, but incorrect use could certainly curtail the beneficial effects.

The first Spectro-Chrome course began on December 7, 1920. At the class, held at 24 East 42nd Street, were 27 students. Among them were two medical doctors, six chiropractors, two dental surgeons and one osteopath. By the time the course concluded several more physicians had joined, bringing the total enrollment to 35. Dinshah taught his students the theoretical and practical aspects of his science and by the end of the course even the laypersons who graduated could "practice" Spectro-Chrome. Graduates received diplomas as Spectro-Chrome Therapists. The course was enthusiastically received and Dinshah was looking ahead. With the $100 tuition each student paid, he could now meet his expenses.

A zealous student in the class, Mae L. Barker, asked Dinshah if he would speak in Philadelphia, her hometown. He consented and she arranged for the Ethical Society to sponsor a lecture there. Dinshah had seen Philadelphia once before — but mostly from the air. In 1919, he flew a plane there carrying the first New York City Police Mail.

With Dinshah's growing reputation and revolutionary claims, he never had difficulty attracting audiences. Often, however, many would come skeptical, only to leave believers, or at the least, accept the possibility of the validity of his work.

In his Philadelphia lecture, Dinshah so completely won over his audience that they unanimously requested an elaborate series of lectures on his science. Dinshah rented space in the Woman's Benefit Building for this purpose and each lecture was filled to capacity.

At the conclusion of the series he was approached by several class members to give a formal course. Dinshah didn't know that one of them, an unassuming woman who gave her name as Kate Baldwin, was the eminent senior surgeon at the country's oldest women's hospital, Woman's Medical College of Philadelphia.

Dinshah told those who approached him at the lecture that he would give a Spectro-Chrome course if there would be at least six students paying $100 each. This requirement was easily met. By the last class on Thursday, June 30, 1921, the enrollment had swelled to 76, including numerous doctors and other professionals from the health field.

In a letter dated June 30, 1921, the second Spectro-Chrome class (including Dr. Kate Baldwin), wrote the following to Dinshah:

We, the undersigned students of the Spectro-Chrome Institute of Philadelphia, PA, completing our course tonight in the Class of Spectro-Chrome Therapy, feel constrained by every sense of gratitude and appreciation, to express many thanks to our noble and worthy Tutor, Colonel Dinshah P. Ghadiali, M.D., who by continuous sacrifices of unselfish devotion to humanity has been imparting to us in 24 discourses with unparalleled zeal by his unique manner, the most valuable general information and practical scientific knowledge of Natural Forces in relation to the mysterious laws that govern Light, Life and Health. Many physicians of this Class, who are graduates from other schools of therapeutics have from time to time witnessed wonderful experiences of the benefits derived from the Attuned Color Waves as used in the art and science of Spectro-Chrome Therapy as originated and taught by Colonel Dinshah, and all of us have heard their reports of satisfaction.

We have enjoyed and received each lesson as an inspiration and a revelation of the Finer Forces of Nature, and explanations and experiments given by this Wise Man of the East have brought into our life new beams of happiness.

We regret the course is over. It seems hard to part even temporarily with the teaching influence of this marvelous Tutor and it is only tempered with the knowledge that in the fall we shall again have the privilege of listening to his orations and to learn more about the great Truths of Transcendental Metaphysics.

We wish Colonel Dinshah the best success in his task of unifying the East and the West, which by his mastery of the Sciences of both the hemispheres and his uncanny sight into human affairs and psychology he is admirably adapted to perform. Finally, we have heartfelt pleasure in commending him to the kindest fellowship of all unbiased and truth-seeking scholars and students.

To avoid the grueling task of commuting to Philadelphia for the classes, Dinshah and his daughter, Kashmira, moved to the city. An office was rented at 1602 Summer Street for $3,000 a year where classes could be conducted.

Soon after, at the suggestion of a student, Dinshah rented a vacant store on Atlantic City's famous Boardwalk and delivered free public lectures. A demand again arose for a course, which he commenced on July 13, 1921, with 40 students, later reaching 69. This class met three times per week and Dinshah found he had a hectic schedule; he traveled 60 miles from his home to each class and another 100 miles each way the next day to New York and home again. But the 48-year-old man had the satisfaction of seeing his brainchild grow.

Word got around of the "curative" powers of Spectro-Chrome and Dinshah was often hired as a "consultant" for people whose conditions were diagnosed as terminal by their physicians. One man wanted Dinshah to go to Baltimore to see his bedridden mother-in-law whose doctor told her she had cancer so far gone that there was no use in operating. Dinshah customarily charged a consulting fee of $1 per minute and the man paid him $600 for the ten-hour trip. But his mother-in-law was soon relieved of pain and two weeks later came to see Dinshah on the Boardwalk.

Dinshah visited Baltimore several more times, giving public lectures. One interested member of one of the audiences was Dr. Arthur B. Bibbins, President of the Maryland Academy of Sciences, who requested Dinshah to speak before the Academy members. Always delighted to lecture on his work to scientific colleagues, Dinshah gratefully accepted.

Dinshah's speech was so enthusiastically received that the Academy invited him to Corporate Membership with the rank of Academician. In appreciation for this opportunity he responded by presenting twelve free scholarships to the Academy to have qualified members investigate his healing science in the fourth Spectro-Chrome class, to be held beginning on October 5, 1921, in Baltimore. On October 11, the Academy granted Dinshah a Certificate as a Life Member and seven months later he was given the rank of Academician for Life.

It had been almost a year-and-a-half since Dinshah mounted a stage in New York City and boldly introduced to the public a healing art he had conceived in his birth nation of India. As he spoke that fateful day, and in his subsequent lectures and classes, always vivid in his mind were the empirical trial-and-error treatments that led him to make such grand pronouncements about his science of color therapy.

He spoke assuredly, maybe even over-confidently, about Spectro-Chrome because he believed the science behind his healing art was incontrovertible. The honors that started to come his way were appreciated, maybe even in his own audaciousness, to be expected. But ever-cognizant of what his healing science could mean to established industries in the health field, potent economic forces that weren't likely to be remonstrated without pulling out all their stops and slaying the enemy, Dinshah accepted the kudos that came his way with calm reserve. Yes, calm reserve. He knew the expression "the calm before the storm" and in anticipating the gales of disparagement to blow his way, he embraced the promise and excitement for his healing therapy that he held on the day he introduced Spectro-Chrome to the world.

2

A SPECTRO-CHROME CHAMPION
FROM THE MEDICAL FIELD

Woman's Hospital, at North College Avenue and 22nd Street in Philadelphia, was established in 1861 as a clinical training facility for students of Women's Medical College of Pennsylvania. Its charter, issued by the Legislature of Pennsylvania, provided for "the establishment in the City of Philadelphia of a hospital for the treatment of diseases of women and children, and for obstetrical cases; furnishing at the same time facilities for clinical instruction of women engaged in the study of medicine, and for the practical training of nurses."

The hospital's origins were embedded in dissent. After the Philadelphia Medical Society prohibited women from joining professional medical groups and educational clinics, Dr. Ann Preston, a graduate of the Female Medical College, later named Women's Medical College of Pennsylvania, rallied a cadre of wealthy women to finance a hospital for the clinical training of female students. The fruits of their labor resulted in Woman's Hospital.

On the surface, it may be regarded that it was a similar gesture of defiance against the establishment, or rather conventional medicine, that Kate Baldwin installed a Spectro-Chrome machine in Woman's

Hospital. But Dr. Baldwin did not implement Spectro-Chome in any manner of revolt but rather in the genuine belief that there may actually be something to Dinshah's unconventional healing art. What, she did not know, but having attended one of his lectures and become intrigued by the possibility of it, as the chief surgeon at Woman's Hospital she had the authority to install the machine, and she planned to use it on minor ailments to see what it could do. After all, when conventional medicine didn't work, what harm could it do? With her extensive credentials she had always prided herself in being scrupulous, but as a scholar of medicine she was also open-minded, even if that meant considering therapies that seemed to go against conventional wisdom.

Not long after Dr. Baldwin boldly installed a Spectro-Chrome machine in Woman's Hospital, Grace Shirlow, an eight-year-old girl from Darby, Pennsylvania, was brought into the emergency room of the hospital, four-fifths of her torso charred, the involved area extending from her neck down to four inches below the groin on her left side. Severely burned when her clothes had caught fire, her skin was destroyed down to the fascia, exposing the muscular tissue.

The attending physician surmised her condition to be terminal and simply wrapped the wounds in cotton and gauze. "There is no use in trying to do anything with this!" he said. The child was put in a special room and several staff surgeons came to look at her. They all concurred that her condition was hopelessly fatal. One doctor who had been in World War I remarked, "Well, we don't try to treat one of those; we give them a big dose of morphine and push them off to the side."

The next day, Dr. Baldwin returned to work, having been out of town on a business trip. Arriving at the hospital she was briefed on the Shirlow case and immediately went to see the girl. The surgeon was horrified to see the extent of the child's burns. What could be done to save her? "There is nothing in traditional medicine to make the child live," Dr. Baldwin concluded. "If she is to live, it will have to be by some other method."

Dinshah's color machine had been set up by Dr. Baldwin in a small room in the hospital. She turned to her assistant and said, "We'll see what Spectro-Chrome will do."

Kate Baldwin did not expect a miracle. Resorting to Spectro-Chrome in this case was simply an act of desperation. She had only been using Spectro-Chrome a short time, and mainly for minor disorders. She had a certain amount of faith in this treatment but wasn't wholeheartedly convinced. In her mind she conceived it could work, and certainly there was nothing to lose by trying it on the dying child.

The girl was moved into the special room. Color rays were normally "tonated" (shined or irradiated) over the body without the affected area being covered. But the cotton and gauze dressing had closely adhered to the raw surface of Grace's skin and could not even be forcefully removed.

Young Grace had a temperature of 105 degrees Fahrenheit. There was complete suppression of her urine output. Fluids had been forced to replete her intravascular volume, without benefit. Forty-eight hours had passed and still no urine.

A Spectro-Chrome "Graduate"-model machine was placed at the bedside of the fading girl. Made of sturdy metal, the electrical, or wired, apparatus with a motor-driven exhaust, had a three-legged base with wheels from which a thick cylinder arose at its center. On the cylinder was an arm that could be raised or lowered so the light could be focused on the patient as desired. The arm was adjustable, which meant it could be extended in or out to also tonate the proper area as required — and hanging from the arm was a projector which housed a 2,000-watt bulb and a blower fan, or breezer, to cool the bulb as it burned when the current was turned on.

At the front of the projector was a slide carrier with two aperture disks on which filters, or color wave slides, could be secured over the apertures; either or both disks could be rotated to give the desired color. There were six filters required. One disk had red, green and violet, and the second disk had red, yellow and blue. Each disk had an opening with no filter so a single filter could be used from either disk. When placed alone or in in different combinations the slides could yield twelve different colors — the red, green, violet, blue and yellow of the disks plus turquoise, indigo, purple, magenta, scarlet, orange, and lemon. Students of Dinshah knew the colors that combinations of the color wave slides could produce. Red and blue yielded scarlet; yellow and violet yielded purple; blue and green yielded turquoise; red and violet yielded magenta; yellow and red yielded orange; violet and blue yielded indigo; and green and yellow yielded lemon.

Dr. Baldwin realized that several colors were indicated in this case. Blue, which is on the ultragreen side of the spectrum, was applied first, since it was known to be effective in relieving tension and pain, especially in burns. The light was shined a few feet away, directly over the dressing. Scarlet light was next tonated over the kidneys at a distance of eighteen inches for 20 minutes, with all other areas covered. Two hours after scarlet irradiation over the kidneys the child voided eight ounces of urine.

Dead tissue had to be removed before new epithelium could grow and so other colors were later applied to promote the separation of the necrotic tissue. At the same time, the doctors paid close attention to the girl's cardiovascular status and kept her on a vegetarian diet in which she was encouraged to drink as much as she could, including natural lemonade made from fresh lemons, water and brown sugar.

To the amazement of Dr. Baldwin and her colleagues, Grace steadily improved, and now a large portion of the original dressing could be removed. To remove the bandages, which had tightly adhered to the damaged epithelium, Dr. Baldwin used colors on the infra-green side of the spectrum such as lemon, yellow and orange. A new dressing, however, was needed to cover the wound to prevent the raw surface from becoming desiccated. A sheet of wax paper and a cloth were put into a sterilizer. The paraffin was removed and a thin, sterilized, absorbent paper was fabricated. This paper was then dipped into a saturated solution of sodium bicarbonate in crude coconut oil. In this manner it would adhere to the dead tissue. For further protection, two thicknesses of gauze were placed on the bed beneath the child and sewn over her, kimono-style. Bandages were not used because their added pressure would have increased the child's discomfort.

During the healing period, nothing was used except Spectro-Chrome — turquoise to build new skin — and a vegetarian diet. Dr. Baldwin was amazed to see the child not only thrive, but, except for slight scarring under the left arm, develop a completely new skin over almost the entire burned section. It was a perfectly flexible, natural skin. At one point one of the nurses remarked, "Dr. Baldwin, you will have difficulty convincing people of the extent of this burn." The chief surgeon agreed but the proof was there. Grace Shirlow, the young girl whom the doctors had assumed would die, was becoming a healthy child once again.

Dr. Baldwin faced an important decision. She was an open-minded physician, but until now had used Spectro-Chrome only on simple, uncomplicated cases. Perhaps it was time to consider its application to more serious disorders — cancer, heart disease and diabetes, to name a few. She could accept the possibility that Spectro-Chrome was everything Dinshah said it to be. But what about her colleagues, the hospital's board of trustees and the American Medical Association? What would they say? Overwhelming obstacles would have to be encountered. Should she jeopardize her 32-year career, seventeen years as the respected senior surgeon of a hospital, to practice a healing science based on light and color which allegedly cured most human ailments?

3

THE SCIENCE OF SPECTRO-CHROME

By 1922 Dinshah had amassed almost 2,000 adherents to Spectro-Chrome including many respected medical doctors. Dinshah had a level-headed business mind and decided to organize his activities more efficiently. He moved his New York office to less expensive quarters at 171 Madison Avenue. In Philadelphia, he purchased a building at 2401 North Broad Street for $30,000 and made this his residence and home office. On the ground floor, he set up a lecture room and secretarial offices. The second floor contained his office and a research laboratory. The next floor had his and his daughter Kashmira's living quarters, and a laundry and balcony were on the fourth floor.

Following his Baltimore class, which he held on October 5, 1921, Dinshah gave another one just six days later, on October 11, but this time in Philadelphia. He was a tireless journeyer because he fervently believed in his healing science and was resolute in his determination to bring it to the masses and alleviate human suffering. Word was spreading in medical circles about this mysterious new treatment called Spectro-Chrome, and Dinshah was bent on making it known to as many professionals as he could reach. Motor transportation in this day was not very swift and not always reliable, but that was not a deterrent to this strong-willed man. Messengers don't mind the inconvenience of arduous physical conveyance as long as they can convey their message.

Subsequent classes were held in Washington, D.C., and New York. In fact, in the span of little more than a year-and-a-half, Dinshah, with equipment in tow, had traversed the central eastern seaboard between these two cities several times. But now he was ready to bring his instruction to a new geographical audience, a Midwestern audience, and on September 20, 1922, after traveling by rail, he held a class at the nine-story McClurg Building, located at 218 South Wabash Avenue in Chicago. With 50 students enrolled, it was his biggest class since his April 1921 Philadelphia group. Dinshah's reputation preceded him and the students were eager to learn about this amazing healing science they had heard so much about.

With the temperature hovering over 60 degrees Fahrenheit on this last day of summer, Dinshah stood before a class of eager students inside the behemoth McClurg, built just before the turn of the century. The class was a heterogeneous mixture of health professionals and laypersons, as usual for a class of Spectro-Chrome, but for Dinshah the only thing that mattered was their interest in learning a new healing method. With such a diverse class, it was always a challenge to present a new science in a way that would be clear to all, not to mention how difficult it was to condense many years of research into one or a handful of classes, but such was his enthusiasm for Spectro-Chrome that he would explain the science in the most lucid and efficient terms he could, and would patiently answer any and all questions from the least-versed student to the most advanced.

After briefly chatting with some of the students, Dinshah stood at the front of the room and took a deep breath before introducing himself. He went through his usual protocol of announcing the richness and excitement of his healing art, and then launched into an explanation of the science.

Spectro-Chrome, Dinshah taught, is the result of the attuned color waves, which are to light and color what music is to sound waves. It is the tuning of the gamut of color waves to rhythmical light oscillations possessing definite influences on the human organism and arranged in accord and harmony with true physical and metaphysical concepts. Its results, he claimed, had been proven under the most severe and rigorous conditions in "hopeless and incurable cases."

The sun is the source of all life and energy on earth, he continued. All growth is dependent on solar energy. Sunlight is transmitted by an oscillatory potentiality of a special character, in which all the elements essential to the chemical existence of the live universe are embodied. From the mineral to the human kingdom, all life is dependent on sunlight. Light is as much a human food (a necessity for existence) as solids, liquids, and gases.

The light evolved from solar energy is white. Its emission polarity has seven main divisions, which can be resolved from it. They are red, orange, yellow, green, blue, indigo, and violet. Every chemical element exhibits a preponderance of one or more of these colors under oscillatory disintegration. The world has all the elements that are known in the sun. The potency of an element depends on the potency of its color waves. Foods and medicines are composed of definite elements and act in strict conformity with such color wave potencies.

Our visible physical body is built of these elements (colors). It contains 72% oxygen, 13.4% carbon, 9.1% hydrogen, and 2.5% nitrogen, which equal 97%. Two additional elements, calcium 1.3% and phosphorus 1.25% equal 99.55%. The balance is composed of all the other elements in the world.

Health is maintained when these elements (colors) are

proportionately balanced. Any disturbance of the element (color) balance is liable to produce a loss of health.

Spectro-Chrome acts upon the physical body, not by absorption or penetration, but by a process of reinforcement or interference on the emanations of the chemical body called the aura or auric vehicle.

Dinshah demonstrated the existence of the aura in his classes. Like an empty pail taking just so much water and then flowing over, Spectro-Chrome Attuned Color Waves are received through the instrumentality of the aura to just such an extent, the excess overflowing into the auric vehicle and dissipating.

Furthermore, Dinshah went on, wrongly attuned color waves will never be received. Were it not for such benign provisions of nature, all photographers working in red light would go wild. Their safety is the aura. As long as one is healthy the aura rejects the excess or uncalled color; when the aura is unbalanced by any disorder, it becomes susceptible to the proper color wave and when irradiated, receives it for normalation.

Spectro-Chrome Therapy can produce similar effects in the bodily organs to those produced by the corresponding drug. For example: yellow is the cathartic (laxative) wave and all drugs producing this effect are found to have this predominant color. However, there is one important difference.

The potency of the Attuned Color Waves is such that it need not be confined locally (for instance a Spectro-Chrome user who tonates one ear could find both ears improve as well as other parts of the body), unlike drugs, which if, say, are introduced into the digestive tract, absorbed and spread through the entire system, affect organs adversely. This idea of color correspondence is applicable also to the food which we eat and drink and the air we breathe. These chemical elements taken into the body are attracted to the various organs, because of the reinforcing relations between substances having similar oscillatory frequencies.

Since a healthy body consists of balanced elements, a disorder, that is to say a disease, occurs from unbalanced chemistry, and when an imbalance occurs it is necessary to correct it to bring the body back to good health again. Poor dietary habits can be the cause of imbalance as foods pervade the body. Therefore, proper nutrition, or foods that do not stress digestion, is recommended.

Dinshah's study of human anatomy and physiology led him to develop a dietary philosophy he called "The Rational Food of Man." It was essentially a vegetarian diet and lifestyle calling for the elimination of alleged harmful substances.

Dinshah found it was necessary to eliminate certain foods which he deemed are injurious to the body and to consume other foods which promote proper nutrition. Fish, fowl, meat, eggs, coffee and tea, he said, can be detrimental — the animal products (fish, fowl and meat) detrimental because humans are non-carnivorous due to their anatomy and physiology as evidenced by their dentition. Humans lack the sharp machete-like teeth of meat-eating animals like lions and tigers and dogs and cats, which can rip sinewy flesh with their incisors. Rather, like the monkey, a fruit - eating animal, humans' upper teeth rest above their lower teeth, or just before it, and are not suited to lacerate sinewy meat. Moreover, unlike carnivorous animals, which can move both their lower and upper jaws, humans can move only their lower jaw, as if it were hinged to their upper maxilla. Eggs should be avoided since, as the menstruation of poultry, they yield toxic gases such as sulphuretted hydrogen which can cause "auto-intoxication." Coffee can be baneful because it has caffeine which can damage the heart and afflict circulation and tannic acid in tea can have an adverse effect on the stomach membrane.

Dinshah identified "Five Essentials" for proper nutrition: bone builders, flesh builders, heat builders, energics, and solvents. Fruits and legumes promote muscular structure; green vegetables with their soft salts cleanse the body; carbohydrates (such as sugar and rice) and hydrocarbons (such as vegetable fats) boost heat; light promotes good health; and water is nature's best solvent.

Dinshah recommended that people avoid artificially-colored and chemically-treated food, lard, white flour, white sugar, white bread and salt (but he said it was okay to eat natural sea salt), and for food to be properly chewed as certainly the stomach cannot carry out that function. He taught it was imperative for food to become alkaline after it is digested prior to it being absorbed into the blood.

The students knew that diet was an important constituent of good health but Dinshah explained his reasoning for all this detail in his work.

Dinshah had divided all of the known elements in his time into twelve colors, and was able to achieve these twelve colors with five attuned color slides. He studied the physiological effects of the various drugs and medicines. Understanding which chemical elements in these drugs predominated, he was able to correlate the positions of such chemical elements on the attuned color wave spectrum.

Every color has its affinity wave which Dinshah defined as attuned color waves which have contrary attributes or qualities of a chemico-physiological character. If there is an excess of color, then the affinity color waves should neutralize it and eliminate the disorder. Opposite affinity colors were lemon and turquoise, yellow and blue, orange and indigo, red and violet, and purple and scarlet. In most cases, Dinshah asserted, pain could be eliminated in one hour. Another example is fever. All fever is caused by an excess of hydrogen (red) and carbon (yellow) and is neutralized by ultragreen colors.

It is the misfortune of the human condition that a litany of diseases, ailments and scourges may infiltrate themselves in the human body, and Dinshah, based on all his research and trial-and-error experiments, described numerous disorders with the appropriate color treatment (his son Darius later catalogued hundreds of disorders in his book *Let There Be Light*). Major and minor disorders alike, his undertaking of color applications to them was encyclopedic. Spectro-Chrome was not a cure-all, he asserted, but nevertheless could be successfully applied to sundry disorders. The conditions he addressed included acromegaly, acute gastroenteritis, Addison's disease, adrenal cancer, acute alcoholism, allergies, anemia, aortic aneurisms, angina pectoris, arteriosclerosis, arthritis, asthma, bad breath, bends, benign tumors, black-eye, bleeding clots, boils, bone fractures, bronchitis, bruises, burns, cancer, canker sores, carbuncles, cataracts, cerebral concussions, cerebral tumors, chickenpox, chills, cigarette smoking, cirrhosis of the liver, colds, colitis, constipation, coughs, cramps, Crohn's disease, cystic fibrosis, cysts, diabetes mellitus, diarrhea, diphtheria, dropsy, chronic drowsiness, dysentery, earaches, eczema, emotional disorders, encephalitis, endometriosis, epilepsy, fibromyalgia, flatulence, food poisoning, flu, gallstones, genital herpes, gingivitis, glaucoma, goiter, headaches, hemorrhoids, hepatitis, hernias, herpes, hiccups, high blood pressure, hysteria, impotence, indigestion, influenza, insect bites, insomnia, jaundice, kidney stones, laryngitis, lead poisoning, leprosy, leukemia, liver cancer, lockjaw, low blood pressure, lupus, macular degeneration, malaria, measles, melancholia, meningitis, menstrual cramps, migraine headaches, mononucleosis, mumps, myopia, neck stiffness, nosebleeds, obesity, osteoporosis, palsy, pancreatic cancer, paralysis, parasites, Parkinson's disease, phlebitis, phobias, piles, pinworms, pneumonia, prostate enlargement, radiation burns, Reynaud's disease, rickets, schizophrenia, scurvy, senile dementia, sex craving, shock, smallpox, sore throat, stomach cancer, stroke, syphilis, tachycardia, tapeworms, teething, tetanus, tics, tinnitus, trembles, typhoid fever, ulcers, varicose veins, vertigo, whooping cough, and yellow fever.

Dinshah surveyed the class of students. Sure, he realized the science could be pedantic to those who heard of the marvels of Spectro-Chrome and just wanted to get on with the business of healing, but before he would let them take that next step, before he would grant them diplomas as certified therapists, he required they learn the theory behind it. Even if these future purveyors of the healing art that he spent many years perfecting didn't need to be scientists to treat themselves or sick people with Spectro-Chrome, he felt it was vital for them to have a basic understanding of the science of Spectro-Chrome in order for them to know it was a bona fide healing system and for them to fend off any challengers. For the challengers, he knew, would come.

4

CASE HISTORIES AND
TESTIMONIALS

By the end of 1922, just two years after he had introduced his new healing art, Dinshah had given nine Spectro-Chrome classes, all except one in close proximity to his home in Philadelphia, in the Mid-Atlantic region of the U.S. The debut New York City class, which graduated in March 1921, was followed by a class in Philadelphia with 61 students graduating in July 1921, Atlantic City with 40 students in September 1921, Baltimore with 46 students in November 1921, Philadelphia with 32 students in January 1922, Washington, D.C. with 20 students in February 1922, New York City with 44 students in June 1922, Chicago with 50 students in October 1922, and Bradford, Pennsylvania with 20 students in December 1922.

Such was the interest in Spectro-Chrome that he created a journal for his healing art and its followers, for, as he wrote in the first issue in June 1922, he had held many classes:

in less than 18 months and the graduates of the Spectro-Chrome Institute spread so widely and produced such beneficial clinical results that they demanded a medium of communication not only among themselves, but between them and the outside world. I bowed to this demand and with this issue, *Spectro-Chrome* sees the light of day to enlighten the world for therapeutic emancipation.

Each month Dinshah planned to diligently publish an issue of the magazine, dispensing information on his healing science, reproducing articles of general interest to readers, offering commentaries on health news and life as well as anecdotes and reports of annual conventions of the American Association of Spectro-Chrome Therapists and Spectro-Chrome groups, and printing case histories and testimonials sent in by health professionals and laypersons.

Many Spectro-Chrome graduates and students had requested an official organ devoted to Spectro-Chrome Therapy so they could learn about the results others had attained with this science in treating various diseases.

After Dinshah decided to publish a monthly journal he went to a local printing company to inquire about rates. Going there in his usual garb and skullcap Dinshah explained the purpose of his visit, only to hear the printer shout to him "I ain't going to print anything for no Jew like you!" Dinshah was astonished, but being dark-skinned he was used to prejudice. He responded in his usual droll way to such crassness. "I am not a Jew," he said, "and if I were I should be in good company because the Benign Lord Jesus was the greatest Jew born!"

Disgusted by the narrow-mindedness of the printer, Dinshah decided that he would set up his own printing plant in the basement of the Spectro-Chrome Institute located at 2401 North Broad Street in Philadelphia. The first issue of *Spectro-Chrome* magazine, published on June 30, 1922, was printed by an outside shop, but Dinshah's presses would be ready to roll by the second issue. With this new publication, Spectro-Chrome, the science, would now be able to reach people in locations where Dinshah hadn't lectured yet.

Dinshah decided to assign a color of the twelve-color Spectro-Chrome system to each issue of the magazine; he framed this by using a six-pointed star, with six of the Spectro-Chome colors in each of the triangular points, and six colors in the interior of the star. The June 1922 issue, Volume 1, Number 1, was assigned the color turquoise so the issue could also be called Turquoise 1922. The July would be designated Blue; August, Indigo; September, Violet; October, Purple; November, Magenta; December, Scarlet; January, Red; February, Orange; March, Yellow; April, Lemon; and May, Green.

In the first issue, Dinshah made it known up front that the magazine would be open to everyone for free expression of opinions, and that the magazine was not proprietary in the individual sense but in the collective sense, just like he wanted his Spectro-Chrome Therapy to be available for practice by all, not just licensed physicians and other health professionals. He wrote in the first issue:

> Although essentially devoted to Spectro-Chrome Therapy, the columns of *Spectro-Chrome* are open to all for exchange of views on everything pertaining to human progress. Its platform is universal and broad in the broadest sense. Spectro-Chrome will be conducted on the principles of an open newspaper owned by the whole world as it were and what none may dare print because of partisan and pusillanimous views, it will publish boldly without prejudice. Its aim will be found to be the most impartial and independent public servant — ungraftable, incorruptible and fearless in the performance of its duty by the exponence of the truth.

Near the front of the inaugural issue was a title page that listed the address of the Spectro-Chrome Institute and brief statements about Spectro-Chrome Therapy: "Devoted to the Latest Revelation in the Healing Art" and "Restoration of the Human Radio-Active and Radio-Emanative Equilibrium (Treatment of Dis-eases) by Attuned Color Waves" and "No Drugs-No Manipulation-No Surgery."

Next, Dinshah's name appeared with the letters of his several honorary degrees, which included: Doctor of Medicine (from the Collegian Medicinae Independentiae in Chicago, Illinois, "Conferred for Thesis on Necrosis of the Bone and for Reputable Medical Practice in Healing by Chromopathy in India," January 30, 1899); Doctor of Philosophy (from Oskaloosa College, Oskaloosa, Iowa, given on June 18, 1912); Master of Electro-Therapeutics (from The National College of Electro-Therapeutics, Lima, Ohio, given on October 4, 1922); Doctor of Food Science (from The National School of Naturopathy, Cedar Rapids, Iowa, given on October 12, 1922); Doctor of Naturopathy (from The National School of Naturopathy, Cedar Rapids, Iowa, given on October 12, 1922); Doctor of Hydrotherapy (from The National School of Naturopathy, given on October 12, 1922); Doctor of Suggesto-Therapy (from The National School of Naturopathy, given on October 12, 1922); Doctor of Chiropractic (from the Nature Science College of Chiropractic, given on October 15, 1920); and Doctor of Optometry (from The National School of Naturopathy, Cedar Rapids, Iowa, given on October 25, 1922).

The first issue of *Spectro-Chrome* contained reports from several medical doctors of their successes with Spectro-Chrome, a miscellany of offbeat and serious medical and human-interest pieces, parables, poetry and letters to the editor. But its most noteworthy component was an article written by Dr. Kate Baldwin. In her article, the chief surgeon at Woman's Hospital described the remarkable case of Grace Shirlow, the eight-year-old girl who was severely burned when her clothes caught fire, as well as write-ups of some other cases Dr. Baldwin had treated with Spectro-Chrome. The article was titled "No Proof of Anything But Results" and, based on the surgeon's actual hands-on experience in using Spectro-Chrome to treat an assortment of medical maladies, effusively praised the healing science.

Dinshah himself responded in the issue to Baldwin's encomium of Spectro-Chrome:

By kind invitation of Dr. Kate W. Baldwin I visited the hospital and saw the burnt girl. It occurred to me that the doctor had certainly produced the most marvelous result in so serious a case. The cocoanut oil and waxed paper dressing was doing all for the application of the Attuned Color Waves through its translucence and the absence of pain to the patient demonstrated the potency of the Spectro-Chrome in the alleviation of suffering which in cases of deep burns is intense, agonizing and pitiably distracting. I congratulate the worthy doctor on her confidence in the power of Attuned Color Waves and exclusively using them against all odds, bravely avoiding morphine and its associates. It is truly hard to believe that drugs could be dispensed with entirely even in such extreme cases and their secondary and tertiary physiological and other adverse effects guarded against for the ultimate complete recovery of the patient. Since the introduction of Spectro-Chrome Therapy into Philadelphia, Penna., about fourteen months ago, the Spectro-Chrome Institute conducted two classes aggregating about 110 students of the system. A majority of these pioneers is practicing in and around the city, but few had such opportunities for clinical observation of the potencies of Spectro-Chrome in such varieties of diseases as Dr. Kate W. Baldwin, owing to her high hospital position, and, without any reflection on the enthusiasm of other practitioners, it might be said that few followed the courses more attentively and put the knowledge to quicker use for suffering humanity than this good doctor. She took the lead to introduce the new system on its own merits under crucial conditions which would have probably discouraged a less competent surgeon, and for and on behalf of the Spectro-Chrome Institute I offer the best and the most beautiful compliments to her. I also convey my sincere thanks to the Board of Managers of the Woman's Hospital of Philadelphia, Penna., for liberal thoughtfulness in introducing Spectro-Chrome Therapy into their institution — setting an example of the nobleness of womankind to the less progressive hospitals conducted by men.

In the same issue were articles by other health professionals. Herbert M. Horn, M.D., D.C., S.C.T., told of how he was seized by a bad case of the grip. He wasn't able to get better on his own and he consulted two physicians and they both prescribed drugs for him. He followed their advice and grew weaker without any improvement in his condition. Then, without mentioning any name, he wrote that:

in our neighborhood there lived a doctor who was considered a faker by everybody. He had certain queer ideas in regard to the treatment of disease. He used to say that drugs were unnecessary for the treatment of disease. He treated his patients with some sort of crazy arrangement of colored lights. But the funniest part of the thing was that the blessed thing worked. This doctor has set right quite a number of people who had been given up as hopeless by the other doctors.

So Dr. Horn sent for this "doctor" (obviously a Spectro-Chrome therapist) and after having had his pulse felt and his temperature taken, was given Spectro-Chrome treatments and ordered to change his diet as told and also to stop taking drugs. "Well, I did as this freak doctor directed," wrote Horn, "and would you believe it, in two days I was perfectly well?"

Alice Norton, D.D.S., wrote about her experiences with Dinshah's healing therapy:

Early in October 1921, I began to use a 400-watt Spectro-Chrome equipment in the treatment of three cases of Pyorrhoea Alveolaris.

The first patient dropped out in three weeks, declaring she could not give the time or observe the dietetic rules.

The second patient, a woman of pronounced dislike for any form of medicine, was interested and willing to be a subject for experiment. She came in the midst of an acute attack, five beautiful anterior teeth being involved (an X-ray examination showed marked disturbance). Removed all calcareous deposits from the necks of the teeth, cleaned and polished crowns of the teeth, and instituted a regular half-hour local treatment of alternate Green and Turquoise in place of the usual routine prophylactic treatment I gave such patients.

There was a marked improvement after the sixth treatment — the patient able to bite apples with comfort — the color of the gums much improved. I then switched to alternate Indigo and Lemon at three-day intervals. I dismissed her after the eighteenth treatment. No recurrence so far.

The third case was a woman 52 years old, a diabetic; she was not satisfactory as a patient, though quite interesting. She is an invalid, comes infrequently, has had seventeen local and two systemic treatments in six months; the improvement was very slight, which is all one could expect under such circumstances. Her physician insists on a "diabetic diet", which includes meat and whiskey! An interesting phase of her treatment is that she always settles herself for a nap as soon as I turn the Green or Turquoise Color on her and she says it rests her for about two days.

Dinshah responded that the cases cited by Dr. Norton:

are interesting and the trouble lies only with the patients or their attending physicians. The patients expect Spectro-Chrome (as a new system) to perform "magic" in all cases without attention to the diet or the technic and rarely give opportunity to the Spectro-Chrome Therapist to show the results by following Nature's laws as indicated. Pyorrhoea should be treated like any other constitutional disease with systemic Green a number of times in conjunction with the local green, etc., and the patient must be patient with the Therapist in going for the necessary treatments.

By this time there were many Spectro-Chrome Institute graduates — health professionals applying the color therapy on sick people and sick people using the therapy on themselves to get better

— and they flooded Dinshah's office with testimonials, either on their own or at Dinshah's invitation.

Each issue of *Spectro-Chrome* contained numerous accounts of cases that reported the propitious results obtained by Spectro-Chrome graduates and students with the color-healing therapy as well as letters of appreciation from Spectro-Chrome classes and endorsements of Spectro-Chrome therapy from classes of students who had completed Spectro-Chrome Therapy training courses.

Here is a small sample of case histories, testimonials and letters that were published in *Spectro-Chrome* magazine through the end of 1923.

∽

August (Indigo) 1922 Mrs. S. G. suffered terribly with piles. Her family physician and others considered her case unamenable and hopeless. She came to me on May 25, scarcely able to walk. I used the yellow wave to keep her bowels regular and the indigo wave on Area 19 [Note: an "area" was Dinshah's nomenclature for a specific part of the body; for example, Area 1 designated the head, Area 4 the left side of the chest, or heart]. Her recovery was so rapid that after her fifteenth treatment she went to Atlantic City where she is still working. A few days ago I met her husband who told me she is doing well. *Submitted by Peter P. John, N.D., S.C.T. [Dinshah noted in the August issue that Peter was "the first Negro graduate of the Spectro-Chrome Institute, a West Indian by birth."]*

∽

September (Violet) 1922 Mr. D., age 37 years, came to me November 29, 1921, with a carbuncle on the back of his neck. He had been treating it for a week or more with the usual home remedies. He was unable to sleep or attend to his usual duties of an interior decorator. Nearly all of the back of the neck and up to the occipital protuberance was involved in the indurated area, but the slough was confined to one side of the median line. There were 24 or more openings in the skin. Aside from the ordinary surgical dressings no treatment was given but the Spectro-Chrome Attuned Colors, which were at first applied twice in 24 hours. The Spectro-Chrome controlled the infection and circumscribed the sloughing area. The skin broke down between three of the openings and the Spectro-Chrome softened and separated the slough so that it was easily removed, leaving a large cavity, which was soon obliterated by the use of the astringent Indigo Wave. It was not more than three days when the cavity was entirely obliterated and the skin soon became normal. The last time I saw Mr. D. the skin was so perfect it was difficult to believe one's own eyes. *Submitted by Kate W. Baldwin, M.D.*

My Esteemed Friend, Dr. Dinshah, Since the day I spent with you in Philadelphia, May 29th, you have been with me, a constant companion of my mind and heart. I owe you a lifelong devotion to the cause you champion ... *Submitted by J. W. King, M.D.*

Dear Doctor, You wish me to tell you what I think of "color light" treatment as perfected by you under the name of Spectro-Chrome Therapy? Let me be brief: for no matter how much I may choose to say, I cannot say more than this: That neither money nor gratitude can pay for what you have given into the hands of the intelligent and conscientious physicians for the *cure* of the ills of humanity. Spectro-Chrome Therapy is not a "cure-all", and you do not claim it as such, but it is one of the most potent means of combating disease and bringing the ailing human body back to its healthy state without substituting one disease for another as it is mostly done under the orthodox method of treatment.

I have used your method and have had excellent results in very serious cases. I am using it now and am having great success, and I shall continue to use it with further good results, I am sure.

I have recently sent to you, of my own accord, reports on several cases, among them two cases of goiter and two cases of chronic eczema, all of which have shown remarkable improvement under the treatment of Spectro-Chrome. I can add now one more interesting case, that of stubborn jaundice of two years' standing. The lady, a widow, has had so far eight treatments of Spectro-Chrome only, and the jaundice has diminished by 50 per cent.

Dear Doctor, I am aware of the immense struggle you are having to break through the hard shell of vanity and prejudice of the M.D., but I am sure you will succeed and that in the end radio-active and radio-emanative forces will prevail over the coarse, sledge-hammer methods of orthodox treatments. *Submitted by Isaac Sossnitz, M.D., New York, New York.*

November (Magenta) 1922 We, the undersigned students, members of the Chicago Class of Spectro-Chrome Therapy, hereby send you our sincere thanks and appreciation. We consider this unprecedented opportunity of instruction and direction from the Originator and Master of so unique a system, of inestimable value. The scholarly discourse on subject touching the deeper and hidden causes of dis-ease have opened our eyes to a greater field of work, and thrilled us to increased effort towards the accomplishment of the real work of the physician — to instruct and lead the sufferer to health.

The personal contact with one who has given so much time, effort and devotion to the task of enlightening despairing humanity, will be to us, individually, and as a class, an inspiration not to be lost with the closing of the class, but to grow upon us as we reflect upon the issues that face us as Spectro-Chrome practitioners. The technical work, covered in the first half of the advanced demonstrations of the closed sessions has been unsurpassed, and, perhaps, as yet beyond our ability to appreciate.

Our humble support and endorsement is hereby added to the increasing force that is gathering about you in the varied activities, including your campaign against obsolete and erroneous systems of therapeutics. *Submitted "On the closing day of the Chicago (Illinois) Class in Spectro-Chrome Therapy, the following testimonial was presented to the Originator of the system. Among the [49] signatories was a number of well-known doctors of medicine, surgeons, osteopaths, chiropractors, naturopaths, electro-therapists and food scientists."*

January (Red) 1923 We the students attending the Course of Instructions in Spectro-Chrome Therapy, December 4, 1922, given us by Colonel Dinshah Ghadiali, M.D., of Philadelphia, PA, fail to find suitable words to express our deep appreciation for the information given us by the Master, in his unique presentation of a science, little understood by the masses which concerns one's welfare in the hour of physical sick-states. We assure you, Dear Dinshah, that the knowledge imparted to us will prove of incalculable benefit to the sick in their hour of suffering and the relief we can give them through your system, Spectro-Chrome Therapy.

Last but not least, we give you double thanks for the information gained in medical and metaphysical lore of which you are a lord indeed!

We wish you God-Speed in spreading the knowledge possessed by you, to impart to others the great gift given us. Man can never reward you for the great work you are doing. We pray that many more years will be spared you at this work. *Submitted by the ninth Spectro-Chrome class at Bradford, Pennsylvania, signed by 19 of the 20 students in the class consisting of 14 medical doctors, two osteopaths, one dental surgeon, and three physicians' assistants.*

~

March (Yellow) 1923 One of my doctor friends is won over to Spectro-Chrome. I shall give this report in the Doctor's own words. "I was taken sick October 3, 1918, with double pneumonia. On October 5th I was taken to the hospital, and was there 18 days. It was just five weeks before I was able to resume my work; had considerable shortness of breath for many months in fact, the bronchial rales have recurred with each fresh cold since. There was an aortic regurgitant murmur, much shortness of breath and for six months had edema of legs; no kidney complications. Since the pneumonia, I have not been able to work as constantly as before and have done my work with less ease; have felt obliged to take at least five weeks of absolute rest each summer.

I took cold the second week in January of this year and for three weeks had a constant cough, so that I was unable to lie down; what sleep I got was sitting up in bed or in a chair. The third week, I think, I did not have more than ten hours of sleep and part of that was with drugs.

The cough was entirely relieved after five Spectro-Chrome treatments. After the first treatment I was able to lie down and sleep naturally most of the night and after the fifth treatment have not coughed at all at night."

Doctor W. is now doing the regular professional work with comparative ease. A neighbor remarked a few mornings ago, "Doctor, you must be feeling pretty well; you walk like a two-year-old" and the reply was "I feel like one". It has been a long time since I saw Dr. W. as well and as happy as at the present time.

Susie T. Age nine years. Had indigestion for a month. On May 22, 1922, there was fever, nausea and vomiting. Pain all over the lower abdomen. Was given Castor Oil; no Bowel movement; pills next day; no bowel movement; pills again before any results. An ice bag on the abdomen continuously. As the child was growing rapidly worse, the doctor in attendance sent her to the Woman's Hospital at

5:30 PM, May 30th. The above is all the history gotten from the family.

I saw the child after her admission to the hospital. The abdomen was distended and very tense. There was evident suffering.

The temperature on admission was 101-2/5 degrees F. Respiration 32; pulse 118. There seemed nothing to do but open the abdomen, which we did at 8:30 that night. The appendix had entirely sloughed; no portion could be found. The right iliac region was full of vile smelling secretion. Everything was a mass of adhesions. To the inner side of the abscess cavity was a mass which looked much like a walled-off fluid. It proved to be the distended bladder which was covered with inflammatory lymph and adherent to the abdominal wall and to the intestines. It reached above the umbilicus and was peeled out as an orange from its skin. The bladder had not been able to contract sufficiently to evacuate the urine.

A twist of China silk was carried to the bottom of the abscess cavity and the wound left open except for a suture top and bottom. Later, these had to be removed. I did not expect the child to live through the night. I wanted to give her the benefit of Spectro-Chrome, but felt that even though no one present expected her to recover, there would be some blame given to Spectro-Chrome if it was used and she died. She *did* live; just why I hardly understand. On the third day, an enema was given and it washed right through and out the abdominal wound. She was too sick to be taken from her bed for any treatment and it seemed each day must be the last. She could not help herself the least. Pneumonia developed in the base of the right lung and there was pleurisy in addition. At this point I commenced Spectro-Chrome, hoping to clear up the lung condition. She was given Lemon, Turquoise, and Magenta. The Lemon and Turquoise given over the whole front of the body. The lung condition responded promptly, the abdominal condition improved and in a few days the bowels were quite normal in action. The nurse remarked, "Dr. Baldwin, we do not have to give Susie any more enemas since you commenced the Spectro-Chrome." The highest temperature was

104 degrees F. The respirations reached 56 and the pulse 148, during the entire sickness.

To the surprise of everyone the child continued to improve and the wound closed. Susie went home October 19th, well, fat and happy. She has reported at the clinic for observation. The last time she came in February and a healthier looking child you will have to go far to find. There is no evidence of there ever having been any abdominal or other trouble, except the scar on the abdomen. What cured the child? Spectro-Chrome. *Submitted by Kate W. Baldwin, M.D., Senior Surgeon, Woman's Hospital, Philadelphia, Pennsylvania.*

The most beautiful result I ever saw is a case of Leutic Conjunctivitis of several years' standing. The eyes were like raw beef. The patient had specialists in numbers, but got no relief until he tried your "light". So, kindly rush me a new bulb. *Submitted by William W. Nuss, M.D., Elkland, Pa.*

Since taking to Spectro-Chrome Therapy in February 1921, I treated successfully several hundred patients. The following are a few of the cases, the full names having been omitted for obvious reasons.

Case 1: Mrs. J. T. Ovaritis. Patient had been flowing for two months. Indigo on 10 and 11 for half hour. Went home well in eight treatments.

Case 2: Mrs. L. S. Diabetes Mellitus. Placed patient on vegetarian diet, but no restriction on starch or sugar. After two and a half months urinalysis shows no sugar.

Case 3: Mrs. A. S. Uterine Fibroid vary large. Almost continuous flowing. Spectro-Chrome Indigo applied daily. Flowing stopped; tumor getting smaller.

Case 4: Mrs. C. W. S. Badly flowing and discharging. Suspected cancer. Indigo on 10 and 11, Green systemic. Flowing and discharge stopped. Patient apparently well.

Case 5: Miss F. Neurasthenia. Patient had been for five years under various treatment without any results. Had been treated by Osteopathy Chiropractic, Electro-Therapy, Christian Science and Drug Therapy, without deriving any benefit whatsoever. Was placed on a vegetarian diet and treated with Lemon systemic. Completely recovered in two months.

Case 6: Mr. W. J. R. Shell-shocked and gassed in war. Respiratory and digestive disturbances. Paralysis of the eighth pair of nerves. Treated with Orange and Purple alternatively on the ears. Orange 4 and 5 Areas, Lemon systemic. Patient is perfectly well.

Case 7: Mrs. S. G. M. Constipation and Autointoxication. Yellow on 9. Patient has daily bowel movement.

Case 8: Dr. W. M. Hepatic hypertrophy. Indigo on 7. Complete recovery.

Case 9: Mrs. B. M. Pulmonary Tuberculosis. Orange on 17, Lemon systemic. Complete recovery.

Case 10: Miss A. K. Anemia. Orange systemic. Patient is well.

Case 11: Mr. E. K. Neurasthenia. Lemon systemic. Four treatments. Condition improved.

Case 12: Mrs. B. F. H. Obesity. Interstitial nephritis. Yellow systemic, Magenta on 18. In five weeks, patient reduced eight inches in waist measurement.

Case 13: Mrs. E. H. Subperitoneal fibroid tumor. Enough size. Continuous flowing. Dyspnoea when walking up steps. Entire system in very poor condition. Main treatment Indigo on 9 and 10. Patient after seven weeks of treatment is in very good health. Tumor reduced to half its size.

Case 14: Mrs. H. G. Continuous inclination to clear the throat. Local examination of the throat did not disclose any pathological condition. Could not diagnose case. Indigo on Area Number 16 and Lemon systemic. Patient is well.

Case 15: Dr. H. M. G. Intestinal stasis. Two treatments of Yellow on 9 cured him.

Case 16: Mr. A. W. G. Eczema. Green on affected parts and systemic. Skin clear in less than two weeks; no itching.

Case 17: Mr. L. A. G. Chronic Gonorrhea. Green systemic and on Area 11. Three weeks now; patient is all right.

Case 18: Mrs. A. C. Uterine fibroid. Indigo on 10 and 11. Four months of treatment. Patient is well.

Case 19: Miss A. B. Uterine fibroid. Two and a half months of treatment. Patient is well. *Submitted by Herbert M. Horn, M.D., D.C., S.C.T.*

The brilliant results of Spectro-Chrome Blue for colds are very interesting. Recently a patient had a noon dental appointment and came with a fresh cold apologizing for the condition as he took the chair. I suggested instead of a filling he should have some "color" for his cold, which he graciously accepted though unfamiliar with the treatment. The history of the case was as follows: Frequent colds lasting two or three weeks with constant discharge; the right nasal cavity and the right maxillary sinuses always involved and painful.

After a treatment of half hour he said he felt better and made an appointment for the following noon. When he reported, he said he must confess that somewhat to his surprise at 7 PM (about six hours after the first treatment) his head cleared and all symptoms of cold disappeared. I related this incident to a young woman, who exclaimed "Good gracious, that beats Christian Science and not half the work!" *Submitted by Delia Riggs, D.D.S., S.C.T., Philadelphia, Pennsylvania.*

I want to report two very interesting cases: Case 1: A Mrs. W., 59

years of age, house wife, came to me on November 23rd, 1922. Her heart was then beating so rapidly and so irregularly it was impossible to count the pulse. She had been treated for about a year by her family physician for Bright's dis-ease, but a urinalysis showed that with the exception of a slight albuminuria her kidneys were O.K.

The last time I examined her this month, her heart was as regular as a grandfather's clock, she could do her housework and climbed stairs without discomfort.

Considering the fact that it was difficult to impress upon her the necessity of adhering strictly to the rational diet and that she was only treated twice a week, her progress was rapid.

Lemon systemic and Magenta on Areas 4 and 18 were the only colors used.

In all my 18 years of practice I saw only two other cases which were anything like it. One of these cases had been treated in the clinics of two of the larger medical colleges in Philadelphia, without the slightest improvement.

Case 2: Miss F. had been treated and mistreated for a period of two years for "colds," "heart trouble," "nerves," etc.; finally, when her condition arrived at the stage of a daily rise in temperature it was diagnosed as Tuberculosis of the lungs.

She consulted me about November 4th, 1922; her pulse rate was 110, her respiration 24. I put her on the rational diet and the lemonade, gave her three treatments of Green systemic and Yellow on 8 and 9 followed by a daily treatment of Orange on 17 and 18 and Magenta on 4.

She has been steadily gaining ground and today she feels like standing on the house top and telling everybody about the wonderful results she obtained from Spectro-Chrome Therapy.

She was examined on Friday last; her pulse rate was 72; her respiration was 16; now her eyes are bright and clear, she is gaining in weight and her whole demeanor indicates a new lease on life. *Submitted by John A. Cohalan, D.O. [Doctor of Osteopathy], S.C.T., Philadelphia, Pennsylvania.*

At the close of this, the Eleventh Spectro-Chrome Therapy course, we whose names are signed below desire to express our deep appreciation to our peerless Master Col. Dinshah P. Ghadiali, for his unfailing courtesy and broad-mindedness. We cannot convey in words our sense of obligation. We earnestly pledge ourselves to apply the knowledge we have here gained to the end that suffering humanity may be benefited thereby, and we extend to Col. Dinshah our heartiest greetings and most sincere thanks for his tireless energy and the world of wisdom he has unfolded to us. May Spectro-Chrome go on to its destined glory to the benefit of mankind and the enlightenment of humanity. *Submitted by the students of the 11th class of Spectro-Chrome, described in the issue as including "two Inspectors form the City of the Department of Health of the City of New York, one former Professor of Chemistry of Columbia University, four Doctors of Medicine, one Electro-Therapist, one Doctor of Chiropractic and several students of law", in a letter dated March 29, 1923.*

We, the students attending the twelfth Course of Instructions in Spectro-Chrome, find that words fail to express our feelings toward our beloved teacher and friend, Colonel Dinshah P. Ghadiali. Little did we realize that 24 discourses could so alter our train of thought and launch us into the great study of the higher side of life. We feel that out Master has put in our possession the most powerful aid to be used in the relief of human sufferings. Every moment spent in the classroom has been enjoyable and profitable and we regret that our course is finished.

On this last day we wish to extend our most sincere thanks for the wonderful opportunities given us and pray that your vision will be fulfilled in the near future. *Submitted by the students of the twelfth class of Spectro-Chrome, described in the issue as "composed of 20 persons, all followers of one or another system of Drugless Healing."*

⁓

April (Lemon) 1923 Among others, I treated the following cases with success:

Case 1: T.C. age 11 years. Ivy Poison on hands. Had three one-half hour treatments in 28 hours; color Indigo. Affected parts dried and healed leaving no scars.

Case 2: Mrs. D.M. age 25 years. Nasal Catarrh of several years standing. Received half-hour treatments every 24 hours for about two weeks. Color Turquoise on Area Number 1. Condition improved from first treatment.

Case 3: Mrs. D.G.R. age 37 years. Severe catarrhal disorder. Received two half-hour treatments in less than six hours. Color Turquoise on Area 1. Result was marked and relieved patient very much.

Case 4: Mrs. E.C. age about 45 years. Acute heart condition. Applied Magenta on Area 4 in two periods of 20 minutes each in 24 hours with very good result.

Case 5: Miss M.M. age 39 years. Chronic bladder infection. Had to be catheterized once and often twice every 24 hours for several months. Applied Indigo on Area 10 every 12 hours in periods of 20 minutes each. After the third day, it was no longer necessary to use the catheter. The patient is steadily improving under correct treatment with Green Systemic, Magenta on Areas 4 and 18, Yellow on Area 9, Indigo on Area 10. She admits she is in better health now than she was during more than twenty years. *Submitted by Gertrude Burgess, D.O., S.C.T., Philadelphia, Pennsylvania.*

⁓

May (Green) 1923 We, the undersigned members of the

Fourteenth Class in the study of Spectro-Chrome Therapy, desire to express to you our appreciation of the extraordinary course of instruction which you have given us during the two weeks which have just passed so quickly.

We feel that the natural forces of the Universe have combined to make you a teacher of unusual power and effectiveness. Your many years of intensive study in the ages-old wisdom of the Orient, combined with your remarkable knowledge of the most modern details in the facts of physical science, have prepared you most splendidly for the great work of teaching humanity the higher knowledge which is so essential to its health and happiness.

But mere knowledge does not in itself make a successful teacher. Your methods of presenting the facts and theories of physics, chemistry and the medical sciences by actual demonstration with the latest types of laboratory apparati entitle you to rank as one of the greatest teachers of times.

The intensive course which you have given us has made us realize as never before the essential unity of the Universe and the basic fact that all natural phenomena are but manifestations of The Universal Energy, a knowledge which will enable us to contribute great wealth of service to the health and happiness of humanity, through the principles and practices of Spectro-Chrome. *Submitted by the students of the Fourteenth Class of Spectro-Chrome, held in Boston, Massachusetts. As noted in the issue of* Spectro-Chrome, *"It was attended by six Doctors of Medicine, five Doctors of Osteopathy, five Doctors of Chiropractic, one Doctor of Magnetism (a graduate of the Institute of Finer Forces established by the renowned Dr. Edwin Babbitt), two Bachelors of Law and Literature, two Doctors of Mechano Therapy, two Doctors of Naturopathy, and a number of others in different walks of life. Several of the students were themselves teachers of various other systems of healing and their unswerving interest in Spectro-Chrome Therapy added to the enthusiasm of the class.*

June (Turquoise) 1923 The following are some of the cases I treated successfully with Spectro-Chrome Therapy:

Case 1: An old woman with chronic varicose ulcer of the foot. Used Purple for two half-hour periods; later Indigo for the pain. In all she had eight treatments; discharged as well.

Case 2: A little boy fell with his chin on some rusty iron which infected the whole lower part of his face, the submaxillary gland enlarged to the size of a walnut and the cervical glands and each side of his neck became very much swollen. I used nothing but the Green Attuned Color Wave over these areas and the abscesses and swelling disappeared. He had in all ten treatments of one-half hour each daily.

Case 3: A woman with chronic nasal catarrh and discharging abscesses that she seemed unable to heal; she was much run down in health. Began with Green alternating with Orange; later used Indigo. To strengthen the circulation I used Magenta over Areas 4 and 18 and alternated with Blue for vitality. She received in all seven treatments of one-half hour each, is feeling well and is singing the praises of Spectro-Chrome Therapy.

I treated other cases with similar success. I feel that all of us who are using Spectro-Chrome Therapy are deeply indebted to its Originator for giving us this splendid weapon with which to fight disease. *Submitted by Charles Rosedale, S.C.T., M.D., Boston, Massachusetts* [*Dinshah responded to this letter in the issue with "I note you place S.C.T. before your title of M.D.; you certainly deserve credit for the foresight — Spectro-Chrome will positively supersede medicine.*]

Mrs. D. When she came to my office she stated the surgeons had refused operation. She was very anaemic and was constantly bleeding so that she had to use several napkins every day in order to keep her clothes from being thoroughly saturated.

An examination showed a far advanced cancerous condition of the uterus, the usual pain and tenderness and bleeding freely on the slightest touch.

I gave her Spectro-Chrome treatment. After the second treatment the flow of blood stopped. After the third treatment, there was no more bleeding and she was able to sleep — which she could not do before — and also to take nourishment. Her improvement was remarkable; so much so that her neighbors remarked a great change in her features and thought it was impossible for any kind of treatment to make the improvement which she showed and expressed themselves in regard to the treatment that it must be something very mysterious.

My honest opinion is that cancerous cases taken before they are very advanced, can be cured, and cases where cure is impossible I feel confident that in every one of these cases the bleeding and discharge can be stopped and the pain relived so that the persons so afflicted will be free from suffering. *Submitted by James Moran, M.D., New York, Member, American Association of Orificial Surgeons, etc.*

December (Scarlet) 1923-1924 Colonel Dinshah P. Ghadiali, Dear Sir, As a representative of the *Oregon Daily Journal* to investigate and report on the merits of Spectro-Chrome Therapy, I beg to report as follows: Personally I might state that I have the College and University degrees of B. Sc. and M.D. and that I have taken a number of Post-Graduate courses. I served for many years as Secretary of the Oregon State Academy of Science.

I have attended every lecture in your Spectro-Chrome Therapy Class and have been constantly impressed with your scientific attainments and clearness of presentation. I have in the past attended lectures by any number of well-known scientists from Huxley down and I feel that your presentation of Spectro-Chrome reveals an understanding of Natural Law that has enabled you to push back the limits of the unknown.

Your fairness, your admiration for all scientific pioneers of the past, indicates a just mind and a generous spirit. Henceforth, Spectro-Chrome Therapy will rank as one of the established sciences and it cannot fail, because it is founded on Truth.

I beg leave to express to you, Sir, my hearty congratulations and wish you every success in your efforts to make this valuable therapeutic agent available to all.

You have permission to use this in any manner as you may wish.

Very respectfully, Ernest Barton, B. Sc., M.D.

Many of the practitioners of Dinshah's healing art, health professionals and laymen graduates of his course alike, reported excellent results with the system. As Wallace F. MacNaughton, M.D., S.C.T., wrote, "The success which has accompanied the use of Spectro-Chrome Therapy since its origination a few years ago is nothing less than phenomenal." But in the September (Violet) 1922 issue of *Spectro-Chrome*, Dinshah noted that some newspapers were warning readers that there were people who referred to themselves as "doctors" when they did not have a license to practice medicine. So Dinshah issued several items to allow those who used Spectro-Chrome to avoid trouble.

Dinshah advised Spectro-Chrome graduates not to call themselves "doctor" unless they had the proper degree; to use "S.C.T." (for Spectro-Chrome Therapist) after their name since they are Spectro-Chrome Institute graduates and the use of these letters is provided by the Institute's charter; to use terms of the Color Wave Predominance System and not those used by surgeons, physicians, osteopaths and other similar health professionals; to not use the word "Disease" since "your patient is at 'Ease'" and "when the said 'Ease' is disturbed there is 'Dis-Ease' so use the word 'dis-ease'"; to refrain from using chemicals or drugs; to refrain from telling patients "you will 'cure'. Man 'treats,' nature 'cures'. You are merely the agent of Nature in this respect and what was induced or produced in your patient by transgressions of Nature's Laws you attempt to remove by rational conditions being resumed. Even in this your methods are far superior to the Drugman's because drugs have their undesirable after-effects; Spectro-Chrome Therapy has no such sequelae:

His final words of advice to those who feared being ridiculed were:

> You, as Spectro-Chrome Therapists, are justified and entitled to your honorable profession of serving humanity and within the nearest future you will be given better recognition by the whole world than is within your dreams today. Back the system and its results will back you; back away from it and somebody will back into you. Act sensibly, for you are not "quacks". A quack is "one who pretends to a knowledge of medicine which he does not possess." Firstly, we do not want or use either "medicines" or what is known as "medical science"; secondly, we know more about the ways in which the "other fellow's" "medicines" act, and thirdly, we discard by very exact mathematical principles the junk foisted on credulous human patients as "medicine" and "medical science" during the last 6,000 years. The term "quack" applies differently now since the introduction of Spectro-Chrome Therapy, and some day unbiased public judgment will uphold the truth. Go ahead! *Get the results, let the public judge.* That will make others quack; for the present, grow on your back a rhinoceros hide topped with a tortoise shell.

5

"THE KING OF DUTY"

The world in the 1870s was on the cusp of revolutionary technological changes. That scientifically prodigious decade would see the invention of the telephone, record player and light bulb, and within the next few decades other exciting new technologies — the motion picture, automobile and airplane — would quickly become part of the tapestry of everyday life. Science was enabling the once unimaginable to become reality.

Mankind's expanding intellectual breadth and soaring ingenuity knew no geographical boundaries. Among the pioneers unfurling the mysteries of science were Thomas Edison in America, Charles Darwin in England, Albert Einstein in Germany, and Louis Pasteur in France.

Bombay in the early 1870s was a lively, burgeoning city in the British-ruled country of India. Its population was quickly growing, it had a venerable institution of higher learning (the University of Bombay), its docks were busy with shipping commerce, and horse-drawn trolleys were just getting underway to provide a public transportation system. Beautiful, bustling and progressive, Bombay in the second half of the nineteenth century was a thriving metropolis where a citizen could find opportunity.

Dinshah Pestanjee Ghadiali was born on Friday, November 28, 1873, at 92 Parsee Bazaar Street in Bombay, India. The first child of Sunabai Pestanji Ghadiali and Pestanji Framji Ghadiali, the newborn, with his wide forehead and coal-black eyes, already bore a resemblance to his father of whom he would later come to be the spitting image.

The baby was not born into any type of royal family. The Ghadialis were of no priestly caste nor were they descendants of a wealthy dynasty. They were a middle-class family and the father was a hard worker and stern disciplinarian.

Under the Parsee system of nomenclature each of the baby's names had the following meanings: Dinshah: "King of Duty"; Pestanjee: "Man with the Holy Body"; and Ghadiali: "Watchmaker" (which was his father's trade). His parents were Orthodox Parsee-Zoroastrians and they would raise their son in their faith.

At the age of two-and-a-half Dinshah began his formal education at Bhulia Mehta's Primary Gujarati School. He was a precocious toddler brimming with energy, and as he got older his restlessness occasionally surfaced in the form of boyish horseplay. Young Dinshah was considered rebellious by his devoutly religious father because he read "forbidden" books and literature about Western sciences, which his father deemed sacrilegious. On August 18, 1881, when he was just eight years old, his discomposed parents sent him to Proprietary High School in Bombay.

Despite his young age, Dinshah, at this new school, excelled in his studies. He studied English in the Fourth Gujarati Class and began to become fluent in the language. He frequented the Cowasji Dinshah Library in the school building and became an avid reader of American science magazines, and these stimulated in him a passion for chemistry.

At the age of nine Dinshah established credit at a local drugstore and purchased various chemicals to conduct scientific experiments.

His introduction to medicine began with an article in *Scientific American* magazine about an ointment of cocaine, chloral, petroleum jelly and menthol that was said to be a cure for headaches. Since his grandmother suffered from severe headaches he whipped up the concoction and plastered her forehead and temples with it, bandaging her head tightly for good measure.

Dinshah once recalled this eventful experience:

> I could barely sleep that night, because of the gleeful excitement in my mind of being the agent of doing such good to my darling grandmother. The next morning, she reported that the headache had totally disappeared. I removed the bandages; the headache was gone, but so was the skin on her forehead. No wonder she loved me since then like poison ivy.

His enraged father confiscated all the chemicals and emptied them into the sewer.

It wasn't long before Dinshah's experiments with chemicals invoked his father's ire yet again. One day he lit some magnesium ribbon causing a huge flare. The tailor who lived downstairs cried out "fire" and a crowd gathered outside thinking there was a blaze inside. When the father heard of this episode he destroyed Dinshah's chemical laboratory and the petrified boy left home. Fearing his son would blow up the house the father signed a warrant for his arrest. The English police found the boy and, charmed by his manner and fluency in English, released him. The father let him return home but once again the fights resumed as Dinshah continued his chemistry experiments. His passion for science was insatiable and he read every book he could find including those on electricity, medicine, light, heat, engineering, and chemistry.

Promoted two classes every six months the lad breezed through high school quickly. He learned English from a multi-volume series book printed in London entitled *Royal Readers*.

Dinshah graduated high school when he was just 11. A

ceremony for student prize-winners was held at Bombay Town Hall on March 22, 1884; it was officiated by the Honorable Justice Bailey and attended by 2,000 people. Young Dinshah received awards for his accomplishments in Religion, Persian, and English.

Dinshah's father was a watchmaker and he wanted his son to follow in his footsteps, but the boy, who had already developed a reputation for being something of a genius, had other interests.

In 1884, when he was a freshly-minted high-school graduate, Dinshah became assistant to Dadabhai Khurshedi Kateli, a Professor of Mathematics and Physics at Wilson College in Bombay. Three years later, when he was fourteen, Dinshah, with Kateli's recommendation, became an experimental demonstrator in physics at seven Bombay academic institutions, although he didn't get paid for his services; soon after, he followed his passion and began the study of medicine.

In early 1891, Dinshah became a member of the India Temperance Society and he began to give public lectures on scientific, religious, metaphysical and occult subjects. On February 10, 1891, he gave a speech at the Framji Cowasji Institute on the value of Edison's new electric lamp, in a speech entitled "Electric Light: Its Production, Practicality, and Cheapness." He was just 17 and even he was surprised that a poor, flimsy teenager — he wore two pairs of pants, one over the other so the holes in each wouldn't show — was now in the distinguished class of scientific lecturers. The 90-minute lecture with numerous experiments, for which he was paid 50 rupees and which drew an audience of 700 people, was sponsored by the Gyan Prasarek Mandali (Society for the Promotion of Knowledge) which had been founded by the renowned champion of Indian freedom, Dadabhai Naoroji.

A year later the boy suffered his first emotional trauma. A girl, Dhunbai, spurned him by instead marrying a wealthy suitor, which caused Dinshah to despair for years.

Friends of the family advised the father to send the boy to England to further his scientific education. He refused and Dinshah, who was known for building electric light installations and was serving as an electrician for his Highness Majaraja Rana Sahib of Dolphur, accepted an offer for the position of Telegraph and Telephone Superintendent for Dolphur State, Central India. He was eighteen years old. Dinshah at this time also began investigating diet and its effects on people and as a result vowed never again to consume meat or alcoholic beverages. He never deviated from these practices throughout his lifetime.

In 1893 Dinshah joined the British Merchant Marine Service and went to work for the Peninsular and Oriental Steamship Company through which he made his first trip to England. The following year he was hired by the Umballa Flour Mills in Punjab, India, as its chief mechanical engineer. He also joined several temperance organizations, including the Royal Artillery Temperance Association under the supervision of Lord Frederick Sleigh Roberts, who had been made Knight Grand Commander of the Order of the Star of India and was commander-in-chief of the British Indian Army. In 1894 Dinshah also served as the electrical engineer to His Highness Maharaja of Patiala.

One of Dinshah's heroes was Alexander Graham Bell, who was credited with inventing the telephone. To publicize his newfangled invention for which he received a patent on March 7, 1876, Bell demonstrated an early prototype at the 1876 Centennial Exhibition in Philadelphia. As Dinshah would later jocundly write about the inventor's experience at the exhibition, when Bell demonstrated the transmission of a person's voice to Emperor Dom Pedro II of Brazil, the emperor dropped the receiver and exclaimed, "My God, it talks!" Keen on the potential of the new communications device, Dinshah lectured on the telephone at the Framji Cowasji Institute on March 5, 1895, drawing a crowd of over 700 people. He was amused that one spectator, at the conclusion of the event, remarked that it was "all bosh! How can a voice go through a copper wire without a hole?"

At this time there were a few dozen spinning and weaving mills in India, most located in Bombay and Ahmedabad, an important city in the western Indian state of Gujarat that was linked by railway to Bombay. The Bombay cotton industry was thriving and Dinshah was hired to install electric light plants in some of the Bombay mills. His reputation growing, Dinshah was made an honorary member of the Poona Volunteer Rifle Corps.

America in the late nineteenth century was the scene of much exciting scientific work and discovery, which prompted Dinshah to visit. He arrived in the U.S. in 1896 at the age of twenty-three, with much ambition but only seventy-five dollars in his pocket. Seeking employment to maintain his sojourn, he met with prejudice. Dinshah was noticeably different. His face, attire and customs were unlike others and he wore a velvet skullcap. One prospective employer called him a "damned Turk" and ordered him out of his office.

Dinshah met some of his greatest scientific heroes while on his first visit to the U.S. These included such illustrious men as Thomas Edison, Mihajlo Pupin, and Nicola Tesla. He visited Edison's laboratory and later spent several hours with him; he also visited Tesla's lab. In fact, he felt a debt of gratitude toward the latter as he later wrote that "I met Tesla in his laboratory at Houston Street, New York in 1896 and he graciously gave me a permit to see the Niagara Falls Power Works." In 1896, Dinshah became the first man in the United States to lecture on the newly discovered X-rays.

Dinshah's reputation in America grew as many newspapers and scientific journals wrote articles about him. The *New York Times* noted that Dinshah was "known in India as the 'Parsee Edison.'" He was highly regarded by many and Princess Viroqua of the Mohawk tribe of American Red Indians adopted the Zoroastrian Indian as a son in a formal ceremony in New York.

Later the same year, Dinshah returned to Bombay and established an obstetrics and gynecology medical practice there. He delivered four hundred and fifty babies and never lost a mother or child. Dinshah scorned the use of forceps, saying the uterus is a woman's best obstetrician. He also became involved in various reform campaigns in his homeland, which were of "radical" character in the hope that they would stir up the people of India.

India experienced one of its worst catastrophes in 1897 when the dreaded bubonic plague ("Black Death") swept the country, killing millions. Dinshah worked day and night in his medical practice and although he treated many patients successfully he felt the terror and horror of this calamity.

One day a young sickly-looking woman visited Dinshah at his office. The woman was passing as much as one hundred motions a day of feces, blood and mucous. Her physician told her that she was suffering from severe mucous colitis and that her condition was hopeless. Drugs had been administered but to no avail. Dinshah recalled a book he had once read, *Principles of Light and Color* written in 1878 by Dr. Edwin Dwight Babbitt, a medical doctor from New York. The book described a method of color therapy using colored bottles, water and light.

Dinshah felt there was nothing to lose by experimenting with color therapy on this patient and after so doing was surprised that she was well enough to resume her daily routine. Little did he know at the start of this experience that he would dedicate his life to the science of color wave healing.

A multi-talented man, Dinshah pursued other endeavors in his free time. He was a skilled composer and a virtuoso musician — he played the sitar, a bowed string instrument known as the Dhiruba, and the reed organ. He was fluent in several languages and appeared on the stage in both dramatic and musical productions. He even served as the stage manager of the Bombay Theater, in which he installed the city's first electric motion picture equipment. Dinshah was awarded an honorary doctorate in medicine in 1899 after he had been practicing for several years; this was customary in India at the time.

Dinshah expanded his medical practice in 1900 when he dedicated the "Electro-Medical Hall" in Ajmer, a large city in the state of Rajasthan, in western India. While continuing his regular medical practice, it was here that he began to treat illnesses by use of color waves and electricity. The following year he opened a similar office in Surat, where his successful treatment of the bubonic plague and other maladies became well known.

In 1902, Dinshah married a Parsee-Hindu girl named Manek (meaning "Ruby") Hormusji Mehta. She was petite and pretty, with large eyes, soft features and a pensive face, and was a member of a temperance organization, the International Order of Good Templars. A year later the couple's first son, Minocheher ("Holy face") was born. Next came a daughter Kashmira, who was born on November 9, 1904 in Surat, India; she was followed by Khushcherer, who was born on June 28, 1906 also in Surat; and then came another boy, who tragically died eleven days after birth.

Dinshah continued his fight against autocratic oppression when he was elected chairman of the Nanpura Parsee Community in 1904. He became involved in the struggle of the poor and often found himself defending their rights in court. This provided valuable experience as Dinshah would later be spending much time in American courts defending himself.

Having been engaged in journalism since 1895, Dinshah continued his interest in publishing when he became a director of the Deshi Mitra Printing Press in 1903. Two years later he founded his own newspaper, an independent and satirical weekly that he called *Impartial* as its mission was to advance freedom of the press. He caused an uproar by exposing political graft and underhanded governmental acts in his column "Our Golden Whip". Metaphysics was also a subject of interest and in 1906 he wrote a book entitled *Himalayi Mahatma Sakramagogo*, or *Master of Occultism*. Dinshah's book was published in the Gujarati language in Surat. By this time, Dinshah was conversant in ten languages, including Sanskrit.

On July 1, 1908 the city of Surat issued Dinshah a Certificate of Identity. The Magistrate wrote: "It is hereby certified that Mr. Dinshah Pestanji Ghadiali, Medical Practitioner, Electrician and

Editor and Proprietor of the Apakshpat newspaper of Surat, is a respectable law-abiding citizen of the city of Surat."

On January 8, 1909, when he was 35, Dinshah and his family boarded the *Caledonia* and left India for a new life. The ship sailed south on the Indian Ocean, continued around the southern tip of Africa, then headed north on the Atlantic. During the voyage, dreams of how his inventions might change the world filled Dinshah's head, which was always brimming with ideas and ways to improve things. The seas were choppy and if that was a metaphor for his future, Dinshah ignored it and was focused on reaching his destination, which was the mother crown of his beloved homeland, the small but historically powerful nation of England. In his native country of India Dinshah had had a variety of avocations including medical practitioner, medical electrician, psychologist, hypnotist, author and lecturer, but in England he hoped to patent and manufacture his electrical inventions, lecture on scientific and metaphysical subjects and study for the bar.

In London Dinshah established the Alcohol-Free Wines Company, Ltd., and set up a factory in Switzerland where he took up the cause of advocating for prohibition. From July 18 to July 24, 1909, the Twelfth International Congress on Alcoholism was held in London and Dinshah attended the conference as a delegate. The Congress's honorary president was Prince Arthur, Duke of Connaught and Strathearn. Dinshah also began to study the relatively new field of aviation and invented an anti-forgery electrical pen, which many English newspapers praised and which the January 22, 1910 issue of *Scientific American* noted that while in the past "such devices have proved commercially impracticable," Dinshah's "simple apparatus" is "very efficient".

During the winter of 1911 Dinshah was in Switzerland on business. It was a brutally cold winter in Europe, and his son Minocheher, who had stayed behind in England, contracted tuberculosis and went to recuperate in a sanitarium. Unfortunately, the sanitarium lacked proper heating, and, exposed to freezing temperatures inside the facility, the boy died. Dinshah carried the boy twelve miles to the crematorium as he was unable to afford transportation and wept as he cremated his son.

Dinshah visited other nearby countries but after three years in Europe of not achieving what he had set out to do, not to mention that his frenetic activities in trying to further the cause of abstinence had caused him major financial losses, he decided to move. He thought his next destination would be Canada, but as it turned out, the country denied his admission. He then set his sights on the country immediately to its south, and on August 9, 1911 Dinshah arrived in the U.S. with the intention of making the country his family's new home; he left behind in London his wife and surviving two children, promising to send for them as soon as he could. It was a time when many people from foreign lands emigrated to the U.S. to flee difficult conditions in their homelands.

In a third wave of emigration that began in 1880, Jews from Poland, Russia, Austria, Hungary, Lithuania, and other Eastern European countries were crossing the ocean in massive numbers to find a better life on the shores of America. Many of these Jews had fled the vicious pogroms of the tsars; they sought a better life in the U.S. and a number would settle in New York City's Lower East Side. For Dinshah, India was under British rule, and that was enough for him to seek the unfettered life he needed to bring his healing science to the public. Like many of the Jews who came before him seeking freedom, he, too, made his first home in the New York City area.

Though he was new to America, Dinshah didn't waste time pursuing professional activities and positions in private commerce. In 1911 he became the chief instructor and examiner in the engineering department at Conty and Company, 485 Park Avenue; an instructor at The New York College of Engineering Science and Automobile Instruction; and private secretary to the superintendent of The Prudential Insurance Company of America, 643/543 West 145th Street.

Over the next few years he held managerial positions at the

Southern Nut and Fruit Company, Independent Electric Supply Company, North Atlantic Metal Corporation, the Union Smelting and Refining Company, and other firms. He was commissioned as a notary public for Bergen County on December 15, 1917.

During these years Dinshah pursued his scientific interests and invented a trolley wire high-tension safety circuit, the "Dinshah Engine Tester" for testing gasoline engines in cars, submarines and airplanes (he presented this invention as a gift to the U.S. Government during World War I although he had been offered a large sum of money for it by a foreign government), and a sound-on-film shutterless and flickerless motion-picture projector. He also started an eponymous company to market and manufacture his inventions. His inventions were written about in numerous New York and New Jersey newspapers. The press also liked to play up Dinshah being foreign-born with a bit of mysticism attached. As *The World Magazine* would refer to him in its July 27, 1919 issue, "He is one of the only and very few Zoroastrian fire-worshippers in America, and is the only Parsee American citizen extant."

On January 22, 1917, after residing in America for six years and having had his wife and two children, Kashmira and Krushcherer, with him for a few years, Dinshah filed a petition for U.S. citizenship in the Common Pleas Court of Bergen County in Hackensack, New Jersey. A Naturalization Officer opposed the application and the judge of the court, William Seufert, asked Dinshah if he was a Hindu or a Mohammedan, because, the judge stated, if he were either he would not be eligible for American citizenship. Dinshah replied that he was neither of those, but that he was a Parsee Zoroastrian. The Court and the Naturalization Office responded that since there was no precedent of a Parsee Zoroastrian being granted citizenship that he should submit an affidavit bearing testament to his being white. Dinshah supplied an "Ethnological Table of the Caucasian Race According to Dr. D. G. Brinton," who in defining the schemes of the races of mankind in classifications based on general ethnological grounds, placed the Indo-Iranic in the North Mediterranean Aryan stock which is in the same group as the Teutonic, Celtic and the Italic nations. Dinshah petitioned that under such classification he was a free white person and was therefore eligible for naturalization. The court received Dinshah's affidavit and turned it over to the Naturalization Officer; naturalization authorities in Washington, D.C. were then consulted. On June 15, 1917, six months after he filed his petition, the court entered a decree for the Parsee Indian to be admitted as a citizen of the U.S. On July 30, 1917, naturalization certificate No. 788770 was issued to Dinshah.

Now a citizen of America, which was emerging as a global superpower, Dinshah himself hoped to find success in this so-called land of opportunity. But as time passed, Dinshah's beloved Manek did not acclimate well to their new country and grew terribly homesick. With his life's mission to introduce a new healing system to the world, Dinshah felt he needed to be in the U.S. and Manek, unable to bear with her longing to be back in India as well as her husband's lack of a steady job and financial struggles, deserted her husband and returned to her native land in 1912. Kashmira and Krushcherer stayed behind with their father. Now his children's sole parent in America, Dinshah hoped to ensure their happiness, but family tragedy struck again on April 12, 1917, when Krushcherer set off an explosion while trying to burn some garbage with gasoline and blew off his fingers and genitals. He died in his father's arms and Dinshah tearfully cremated his second child.

In 1918 Dinshah was commissioned as a Surgeon Captain in the New York Police Reserve (his appointment letter from Inspector John F. Dwyer cited the New York City Police Department's "reposing special trust and confidence in the Patriotism, Valor, Fidelity and Abilities of Dinshah P. Ghadiali"), and in 1919 he became Governor of the Police Aviation School. He organized the Flying Police, an aviation branch of the New York Police where for free he trained pilots, and he was commissioned Colonel of the New York Police Reserve Air Service. For the rest of his life people addressed him with this title. Dinshah flew the first Police Air Mail from New York to Philadelphia and was commander of the Police Air Reserve Service. When the American World War I hero General John J. Pershing returned to New York, Dinshah was in charge of the police boat that received him. For his exemplary service to the Police Department of New York, he received the bronze "Liberty Medal" from Mayor John F. Hylan of New York City. The Colonel retired from the Air Service later in 1919.

Dinshah was even a bit of a woman's rights champion in these days before the Nineteenth Amendment to the U.S. Constitution, which in 1920 granted women a right they previously did not have — the right to vote. According to the July 18, 1919 issue of the *New York Times*, at a conference of the National Association of Drugless Physicians in Atlantic City, Dinshah "voiced a protest ... against Atlantic City's beach law compelling all women in bathing raiment to wear stockings." At the convention more than half the attendees were women. "Why should beautiful women," Dinshah said, "and all the women I see here are beautiful, be compelled by an unmoral, un-American, and inhumane law to cover their beautiful limbs?" The women erupted in applause. "What is the difference, I ask you, between a woman's foot and a man's foot? Do not the authorities yet know that they cannot make people moral by law, that only education can do that? Why not make men wear stockings upon legs that are not beautiful and put all horses in trousers? If Atlantic City would be truly moral it would tell women to discard their clothing or don trousers. I hold she has that right no less than man."

During these years, Dinshah had devoted much time to his medical interests. He joined the American Association of Progressive Medicine in 1918 and served as vice-president of the Allied Medical Association of America and the National Association of Drugless Practitioners.

With his grandiose vision, Dinshah wanted to alleviate the suffering of humankind. A kind and benevolent person, he had founded numerous charities for Parsees as well as others of a more general nature in India, and in 1893 established a hospital. He knew first-hand the fragility of life and the perniciousness of disease. But despite his own personal tragedies, Dinshah pursued life with zest and vigor. He was that rare breed of intellect and charismatic character who electrified people he met and left a lasting impression upon them. While always busy with commercial pursuits to pay bills and provide necessities for his family, he was also all this time deeply involved in independent research. And so in 1920, when he was drawing $15,000 a year from his various business enterprises, he resigned from his positions because he believed he had finally perfected and completed a healing science and was ready to introduce it to the world.

6

MARRIAGE IN THE U.S.

Dinshah was easily able to acclimate to American society, although the reverse wasn't true. He may have been a citizen of the U.S. by now but his looks belied it. Small in stature, with dark skin and narrow eyes, and accustomed to dressing in the garb of his native country, Dinshah still very much looked like a foreigner. America may have been a world power and people had the chance to strike it rich there, as the cliché of immigrants went, but many of its citizens didn't take kindly to those who didn't look like they were born there.

When it came to romantic relationships in the America of the teens and 1920s, liaisons followed a strict protocol of propriety: men betrothed women, and romantic liaisons of all other kinds occurred strictly between members of their own groups. Anti-miscegenation laws were still on the books in some states forbidding marriage or sexual relations between all sorts of disparate groups including combinations of white, African, Asian and Native American people.

A few years after he became a U.S. citizen, Dinshah entered into a romantic relationship with an American woman of white parents and German descent. She was Irene Grace Hoger, born on December 1, 1904 at 43 William Street in Orange, New Jersey. Her father had worked for the renowned American inventor, Thomas Alva Edison.

Irene, raised with no religious faith, wrote in a religious induction document that she "became acquainted with Dinshah Peshotan Ghadilai in the spring of 1921 through the humanitarian work he was doing and thereafter through my constant association with him in his Spectro-Chrome Metry Institute, was highly impressed with the purity and excellence of the Sacred Doctrines of Zararhushtra, whose tenets he followed in daily life."

Dinshah and Irene Grace Hoger married on March 14, 1923. As Dinshah would write about her in the March (Yellow) 1923 issue of *Spectro-Chrome*:

> She was my daughter's companion and my personal secretary during 18 months prior and displayed during that period such remarkable faithfulness and loyalty to duties, such truthfulness and zeal, such extraordinary aptitude for any line of work she was given and without ostentation sank so quietly into the intensive public work I was doing, that I could not remain unsusceptible to the great Karmic link that was forging in the chain of my incarnation. It was she who drew the sketch of the Birth of Spectro-Chrome in the first issue (June 1922) of *Spectro-Chrome* and her simplicity in dress, non-following of the foolish fashions, avoidance in totality of paints, powders, fluffs, frills and frumpery so dear to the average flapper were so to my liking that I seriously began to consider her absorption into my life's career. Her devotion to the cause of humanity through Spectro-Chrome Therapy and her working with me through the same long hours of strenuousness drew her daily closer to me, until, finally when she agreed to take to the tenets of my Orthodox Zoroastrian Faith and began to practice them daily in life, I proposed marriage to her one morning, went promptly to the Philadelphia City Hall, secured the license with the consent of her guardian (she being an orphan) and were married the same afternoon by Magistrate Dennis F. Fitzgerald, without any fuss,

ceremonial farce, false expense or foolish paraphernalia. Not a gift was given or exchanged in either side — not even the customary wedding ring, the eternal representative of human slavery. God is a circle whose centre is everywhere and whose circumference is nowhere to be found. We carry Him in our heart and honest just dealings with fellow human beings and on this entrance into what is commonly called the highest bond, I exemplified my preachings of simple life by shunning all worldly stupid demonstrations. Our wedding was on a working day (we filed the many income tax reports of Spectro-Chrome Institute that night) and our honeymoon was begun with work, more work and service to humanity — and we feel happier for it. It was a marriage of 49 to 18, but even my daughter Kashmira believes it right, so that settles the question!!!

In the same issue of *Spectro-Chrome*, Irene Grace Dinshah penned an essay entitled "Why I Married Dinshah":

When the originator of Spectro-Chrome Therapy, Colonel Dinshah P. Ghadiali took Philadelphia, Pennsylvania by storm in February 1921, we were quite unprepared for his whirlwind methods; yet, we admired his fearless ways.

The first time I had the pleasure of hearing Dinshah orate was two years ago, in the Spring of 1921 at Witherspoon Hall, Philadelphia, Pa., where admiration for his genius and his work was aroused in me. We are merely existing, thought I; it has taken this man to come and teach us what life really is.

While he was bombarding the public by his straightforwardness, little did he realize that he was soon to bombard my poor little heart with the Magenta Wave also!

In September 1921, I attended one of Dinshah's lectures at Atlantic City, New Jersey and at his request (which had been my secret wish for months previous), I joined his activities and launched into the uplifting work of Spectro-Chrome Therapy, which, in my estimation, is one of the greater and nobler works man has originated for his fellowmen.

Those who call this man (who is now my husband) "strict, harsh and heartless," forget that he leads a peculiarly multiple life, so to speak — as an occultist, researcher, teacher, commercializer and family man combined.

Dinshah of private life is entirely a different man from the public Dinshah. The thunderer of the platform, the disciplinarian of the classroom, the merciless harsh critic and satirist transform into an exceedingly human, gentle-hearted big boy bubbling with the vigor of a quick and impulsive mentality, ultra-affectionate heart and the physical animation of a true playmate and companion of joys and sorrows. This side of his life is even visible at times to an audience attuned to his frank and open methods. I wish the World could see him always as I see him in the home. It was *that* Dinshah whom I had the exceptional opportunity of visualizing every day for nearly eighteen months and it was that man who attracted me. What Dinshah teaches as the value of good thought, kind deeds and noble actions he exemplifies: to him they have become second nature. His home life is marked by the most rigid simplicity; he dislikes artificialities and worships the Truth; it was all that which drew me to him. Although a bold lion-like lecturer, he is a lamb-like lover.

I had determined to marry a loving, clean-cut, brainy man and (having learned the advantages) upholding vegetarian diet, that meant one more necessary point added to my already elongated qualifications desired in a soul-mate. It has been repeatedly mentioned that girls always manage to "get their own way" and I have no reason whatsoever to doubt that assertion, because I attained my ideal.

I know Dinshah and his virtues — I also know his limitations as a human being. He is contented and so am I. We are happy in the one thought that we shall both serve humanity with one purpose and aim and shall be of services to those who need our assistance.

The great door of sympathy opened when I knew Dinshah's life was not all roses, but that countless thorns filled the years of unselfish toil — the sorrowful life he has undergone so that eventually suffering humanity might be benefitted: And as sympathy and self-sacrifice are the roots to love, when they sprouted we married and are going to be — "happy ever after".

Religion was ingrained in Dinshah at an early age, having come from a family in which Zoroastrian religion was an inextricable part of their heritage. A man of science, Dinshah saw no conflict in belief in a higher power and a world in which logical, deductive and precise rules applied. As he grew older, and came to know the wonders and strictures of science, his faith never wavered one bit.

Dinshah apparently diverged from the customs of his faith when he converted his wife and daughter to Zoroastrianism. He was from an upper-class family but not from a priestly caste, in which case he would have been allowed to perform the sacred Navjote (initiation) ceremony into the Zoroastrian religion on a boy under the age of twelve, and a girl under the age of seven. However, some explanation for his conducting the conversion may be gleaned from a later writing, in which he stated the he performed the ceremony "in the absence of any Zoroastrian Mobed (Minister) in America; even if there were such Minister of the Zoroastrian Faith, the parents would not have permitted him to perform the sacred Occult Ceremony unless the Minister too were a total Abstainer and Vegetarian in conformity with the strict principles followed by the entire family, such is their rigidity."

On the morning of November 15, 1923, Dinshah performed the Navjote ceremony on his wife Irene and his daughter Kashmira at their residence at 2401 North Broad Street in Philadelphia. Kashmira was born "of white Parsee Zoroastrian parents," she wrote in her induction deposition, on November 9, 1904 "in the Electro-Medical Hall, Maccai Bridge, City of Surat, Presidency of Bombay,

India." Even though her father had educated her in Zoroastrian teachings, Kashmira had never been inducted into the religion.

The Navjote ceremony is used to induct people into the Zoroastrian religion, and in the ceremony they may begin to wear the religion's attire. There are two elements to the raiment: the sedreh, a garment worn underneath outer clothing which is supposed to ward off evil spirits, and the Kushti, a girdle tied around the waist composed of six dozen threads symbolizing the chapters of the religion's formal assemblage of doctrines called the Yasna.

Prior to the ceremony the inductees take a "nahan", or ceremonial bath, in a nearby bathroom. There is also a spiritual cleansing referred to as a "nirangdin" in which the inductee chants prayers and crunches a pomegranate leaf. The ritual also includes wearing other special garments and a ceremonial walk.

Dinshah noted that he performed the ceremony in strict accordance with the Holy Zend Avesta's precepts, except for the ritual of the "Pomegranate for the customary Nerang". Both his wife and daughter, he wrote, were "invested ... with the Sudreh and Kushti, the potential occult emblems of the religion of the Glorious Lord Zarathushtra, the Prophet of Ancient Iran, initiating them into the faith of my revered ancestors."

Dinshah and his wife and daughter signed a deposition relating to the induction, and it was signed by two notaries public.

Dinshah was methodical in everything he did. A prolific writer, he recorded his thoughts and deeds meticulously. The ordination was made, he wrote, "in accordance with my firm belief and teaching that conscience alone is the justification for admission into a faith."

7

AN ARTICLE IS PUBLISHED AND THE "COLOR WAR" BEGINS

With her success in the Grace Shirlow case, Dr. Kate Baldwin decided to add three more Spectro-Chrome machines to bring the total to four in Woman's Hospital. She knew installing the first machine was a radical move, but with her own success and that of other physicians and health professionals across the country reporting excellent results with colored-light healing she was sanguine about her prospects of convincing others that the therapy was not only beneficial, but perhaps even a new front in medicine.

Though some may have inwardly questioned Baldwin's decision, her credentials were beyond reproach: she was the senior surgeon of one of the country's most distinguished hospitals, a Fellow of the American Academy of Ophthalmology and Oto-Laryngology, a member of the American College of Surgeons, a Life Member of the Maryland Academy of Sciences, and a member of the County and State Medical Societies in Pennsylvania, New York and Rhode Island.

With four machines in the hospital, Baldwin took upon herself the objective of more actively treating sick people by shining colored lights on them. Even though she was pleased with the results of

Spectro-Chrome in the hospital in sundry cases, she anticipated negative reaction to her decision so she asked if she could appear before the Hospital's Board of Managers to discuss the new healing science she had implemented there. Spectro-Chrome had been in daily use at the hospital and by the end of 1922 the hospital's senior surgeon had used it in over 300 cases, most of them serious. The Board held regular meetings and on December 21, 1923 Dr. Baldwin was granted an appearance. There were 20 managers present, including the Chair, Miss Saunders.

With her customary poise, Dr. Baldwin described the excellent work being done in the hospital with Spectro-Chrome. She described in detail the case of the young girl Grace Shirlow whom she said would have succumbed to her injuries were it not for Spectro-Chrome. The girl was brought into the meeting room and undressed so the managers could examine the large area that had healed. Anything outside of conventional medicine would customarily be regarded by hospital boards as quackery, but the board was so impressed by the results that it suggested the case be written up for publication. In the minutes it was recorded: "The Spectro-Chrome is used in no other hospital and great credit should be given to Dr. Baldwin for developing its use here."

As colored-light healing in general would undoubtedly be frowned upon by the medical establishment, not to mention that Dinshah's Spectro-Chrome would invite the wrath of organized medicine since it largely removed the need for licensed medical doctors, sure enough, trouble was soon to come for Dr. Baldwin.

On January 26, 1924 the American Medical Association published a scathing three-page article in its *Journal* (*JAMA*) ridiculing Spectro-Chrome and excoriating Dinshah (ironically, the article following Dinshah and Spectro-Chrome in *JAMA* was titled "Some New Lines of Progress In Cancer Research").

Preceding the article was a brief note explaining its raison d'être: a request by a Dr. Harry J. Powers of Los Angeles, "one of the many correspondents to inquire about the fearfully and wonderfully named

Dinshah P. Ghadiali and his 'Institute' and 'Therapy'," for "a word about the Spectro-Chrome Institute".

The article then commenced with unceremonious scorn:

Nothing pays so well nowadays as floating a new freak therapy. If the thing is worked with finesse and plausibility, the public will "eat it up". Moreover, venal ignoramuses in the various drug cults will espouse with enthusiasm any new "system" that is widely advertised and can be practiced without violating the Medical Practice Acts of the various states.

After listing some past practitioners of color therapy, the article stated: "now comes into the field Colonel Dinshah P. Ghadiali." It said he had "an appalling list of titles", including "that of M.D.," and that the records of the AMA indicated that "no man by the name of Dinshah P. Ghadiali has ever been graduated by any reputable medical college nor licensed to practice medicine in any state of the Union."

The article went on to cynically relate Dinshah's biography and with the same derisive tone then describe the science behind Spectro-Chrome Therapy. The section on the science ended with this:

"Spectro-Chrome Therapy," says Ghadiali, will "meet every condition of ill health." Like our friends the Eddyites, however, he recognizes and admits the limitation of his therapy in surgical cases. As all the Colonel's pictures show him wearing spectacles, one presumes also that "attuned color waves" are valueless for correcting errors of refraction.

The next section of the article chastised Dinshah's take on drugs, quoting him as saying they "quickly upset the nervo-vital balance of persons of high mental and spiritual development." Thus "the mental and spiritual high-brow who is feeling off-color should therefore, purchase the 'Standard Spectro-Chrome outfit'" which can be purchased directly from Dinshah himself.

In this way, the article proclaimed, did Dinshah "appeal to that vast field, the hypochondriac public," attempting to engage "with equal plausibility medical men and the followers of the so-called 'drugless cults'." It then related that Dinshah traveled the country to give courses on Spectro-Chrome Therapy, charging students $100 and requiring them to sign a statement that "they will never give out, print, or publish, either directly or indirectly, any of the notes taken during the course, nor any part of the 'instructions, charts, diagrams, processes and the like.'" Then the "disciple" gets a diploma and "is permitted to call himself a 'Spectro-Chrome Therapist' and put after his name the magic letters 'S.C.T.'"

Dinshah's business practices were next criticized in the article: "We learn that 'bulbs, charts and similar supplies maybe had for cash' and Ghadiali emphasizes that his institute does not maintain a credit department, that all transactions are net cash with order and the Institute's responsibility ceases with shipment."

Personal checks are acceptable but orders will not be shipped until the checks clear.

The final section on "Testimonials" crescendoed in disparagement, making its new target the medical doctors who allegedly obtained excellent results with Dinshah's science. "Like every cult of any pretensions," the section began, "'Spectro-Chrome Therapy' has a house-organ." The publication, *Spectro-Chrome*, "contains the usual number of testimonials and these are funny or very tragic, according to the way you look at them." It then denigrated Dr. Kate Baldwin, who wrote in the March 1923 issue of *Spectro-Chrome* about a nine-year-old patient who "was admitted to the Woman's Hospital with a sloughed appendix and peritonitis" and "developed pneumonia". Poking fun at Dr. Baldwin who treated the girl with turquoise, magenta and lemon lights, it quoted Dr. Baldwin as saying "Susie went home ... well, fat and happy."

Other successful case histories with Spectro-Chrome were then related before the article concluded:

> A cult to be successful must have plausibility. It should have some apparent scientific basis. The Spectro-Chrome fad plays on the public's ignorance of light therapy ... What more plausible, then, to those possessing that small knowledge that is dangerous, that human pathology is due to a lack of balance in the alleged 'color wave potencies' — whatever that may mean.

Some physicians, after reading this article, may wonder why we have devoted the amount of space to a subject that, on its face seems so preposterous as to condemn itself.

When it is realized that helpless but credulous patients are being treated for such serious conditions as syphilitic conjunctivitis, ovaritis, diabetes mellitus, pulmonary tuberculosis and chronic gonorrhea with colored lights, the space devoted to this latest cult will not be deemed excessive.

In response to the pejorative AMA article — which essentially ignited a "color war" between the originator and followers of Spectro-Chrome and the organized forces of professional medicine — Dinshah sent a cordial letter to the *Journal* editor on February 24 asking for an investigation of his healing science and pledging to send advance funds to facilitate the research. Two months passed by without a response so Dinshah wrote the editor again, this time enclosing with his letter the October 1923 issue of *Spectro-Chrome* which contained a report of the case the *Journal* covered. Still, no response. And so, two months later, on June 2, Dinshah sent to the AMA's Executive Council a telegraph once again cordially asking for an investigation of his system. There was no response to the telegraph yet further denunciations about him persisted and so on September 22 he openly challenged the AMA to publicly debate Spectro-Chrome, and by his own behest included a self-imposed penalty against himself:

If you win, I am willing and ready to present to you all my inventions, patents, copyrights, trademarks, business, printing plant, processes for manufacture— everything I have including my entire Spectro-Chrome Institute and all its belongings, give you an abject unconditional apology and forever retire, leaving the country never to return.

There was no response to Dinshah's open challenge. (Without any acknowledgment whatsoever over the years, the AMA's impudence was not lost on the devoted followers of Spectro-Chrome. On November 10, 1934, at the 14th Annual Convention of the Healing Science which was attended by 1,000 people at the Milwaukee Auditorium in the Wisconsin capital, a unanimous resolution was passed in which by not accepting or taking part in the challenge the recipients, that is, the AMA, "branded themselves as liars and cowards.")

The AMA article talked in generalities and didn't address any of the specific cases in which health professionals used Spectro-Chrome with reportedly successful results. As Dr. Baldwin wrote in the first issue of *Spectro-Chrome* in an article titled "No Proof of Anything But Results":

A statement of opinion is as nothing compared with a report of experience. Repeated successes allow of no other conclusion than that experience with Spectro-Chrome Therapy or Attuned Color Waves has proved its value. This truth is worthy of all reiteration it can be given.

Here I can only mention in a general way some of the results secured by the use of Attuned Color as a therapeutic measure. It is the most well-worth-while contribution to the healing art in many years. I doubt if anything known to "scientific medicine" can show more satisfactory results.

After the *Journal* article was published, the staff at Woman's

Hospital requested the board ask Dr. Baldwin to stop using Spectro-Chrome as a healing therapy. According to the Board minutes of March 28, 1924, "The matter of asking Dr. Baldwin to discontinue the use of Spectro-Chrome Therapy was left to a committee composed of Mrs. Shoemaker, chairman, Mrs. Stone and Mrs. Tatum." A month later the minutes announced "Mrs. Shoemaker reported progress on the Spectro-Chrome Therapy and this matter was left in the hands of the committee for a further report in May..." The minutes of May 24, 1924 stated "Mrs. Shoemaker, for the Committee to investigate the Spectro-Chrome Therapy, said that the question had been considered from every viewpoint and that the Committee recommended the continuance of present conditions. This report of the Committee was accepted."

It would seem this was a victory for Spectro-Chrome and Dr. Baldwin, and that she would be able to carry on her efficacious practice of light therapy at the hospital. Indeed, on March 27, 1925, the minutes reported: "Dr. Baldwin in a letter spoke of her need of more room for the Spectro-chrome. She asked to have two cubicles made; she is getting many cases and needs more room. Mrs. Shoemaker moved that this matter be left with the Clinics Committee. Motion carried. Miss Plumer moved that the Clinics Committee also have the power to act. Motion carried."

If Spectro-Chrome wasn't deemed to have been working as a healing art the board surely would have discontinued its use in the hospital. But the *Journal* article did its damage and the hammer was soon to fall.

The minutes of September 24, 1926 stated:

Letter from the Internes, objecting to Dr. Baldwin's presence on the Surgical Staff. Mrs. Earle moved that the Board of Managers request Dr. Baldwin's resignation from the Surgical Staff, if such request meets the approval of the majority of the General Staff and that Dr. Baldwin be granted the privilege of practicing Spectro-

Chrome Therapy with her private patients in the Woman's Hospital. This motion was seconded and carried.

On October 12, 1926 Kate Baldwin presented a paper at a clinical meeting of the Medical Society of the State of Pennsylvania's Eye, Ear, Nose and Throat Diseases section. It was to become a fundamental doctrine in support of Spectro-Chrome. Here is Dr. Baldwin's paper, which was reprinted in the April 1927 issue of *Atlantic Medical Journal*:

The Therapeutic Value of Light and Color

In the effort to obtain relief from suffering, many of the more simple but potent measures have been overlooked while we have grasped at the obscure and complicated.

Sunlight is the basic source of all life and energy upon earth. Deprive plant or animal life of light, and it soon shows the lack and ceases to develop. Place a seed in the very best of soil or a human being in a palace, shut out the light, and what happens? Without food (in the usual sense of the term) man can live many days; without liquids a much shorter time; but not all without the atmosphere which surrounds him at all times and to which he pays so little attention. The forces on which life mostly depends are placed nearly or quite beyond personal control.

For centuries scientists have devoted untiring effort to discover means for the relief or cure of human ills and restoration of the normal functions. Yet in neglected light and color there is a potency far beyond that of drugs and serums.

In order that the whole body may function perfectly, each organ must be one hundred percent perfect. When the spleen, the liver, or any other organ falls below normal, it simply means that the body laboratories have not provided the required materials with which to work, either because they are not functioning as a result of some disorder of the internal mechanism, or because they have not been provided with the necessary materials. Before the body can appropriate the required elements, they must be separated from the waste matter. Each element gives off a characteristic color wave. The prevailing color wave of hydrogen is red, and that of oxygen is blue, and each element in turn gives off its own special color wave. Sunlight, as it is received by the body, is split into the prismatic colors and their combinations as white light is split into the prismatic colors and their combinations as white light is split by passage through a prism. Everything on the red side of the spectrum is more or less stimulating, while the blue is sedative. There are many shades of each color, and each is produced by a little different wave length. Just as sound waves are tuned to each other and produce harmony or discords, so color waves may be tuned, and only so can they be depended on always to produce the same results.

If one requires a dose of castor oil, he does not go to a drug-store and request a little portion from each bottle on the shelves. I see no virtue, then, in the use of the whole white light as a therapeutic measure when the different colors can give what is required without taxing the body to rid itself of that for which it has no use, and which may do more or less harm. If the body is sick it should be restored with the least possible effort. There is no more accurate or easier way than by giving the color representing the lacking elements, and the body will, through the radioactive forces [the aura], appropriate them and so restore the normal balance. Color is the simplest and most accurate therapeutic measure yet developed.

For about six years I have given close attention to the action of colors in restoring the body functions, and I am perfectly honest in saying that, after nearly thirty-seven years of active hospital and private practice in medicine and surgery, I can produce quicker and more accurate results with colors than with any or all other methods combined — and with less strain on the patient. In many cases, the functions have been restored after the classical remedies have failed. Of course, surgery is necessary in some cases, but the results will be quicker and better if color is used before and after operation. Sprains, bruises and traumata of all sorts respond to color as to no other treatment. Septic conditions yield, regardless of the specific organism. Cardiac lesions, asthma, hay fever, pneumonia, inflammatory conditions of the eyes, corneal ulcers, glaucoma, and cataracts are relieved by the treatment.

The treatment of carbuncles with color is easy compared to the classical methods. One woman with a carbuncle involving the back of the neck from mastoid to mastoid, and from occipital ridge to the first dorsal vertebra, came under color therapy after ten days of the very best of attention. From the first day of color application, no opiates, not even sedatives, were required. This patient was saved much suffering, and she has little scar.

The use of color in the treatment of burns is well worth investigating by every member of the profession. In such cases the burning sensation caused by the destructive forces may be counteracted in from twenty to thirty minutes, and it does not return. True burns are caused by the destructive action of the red side of the spectrum, hydrogen predominating. Apply oxygen by the use of the blue side of the spectrum, and much will be done to relieve the nervous strain, the healing processes are rapid, and the resulting tissues soft and flexible.

In very extensive burns in a child of eight years of age there was almost complete suppression of urine for more than forty-eight hours, with a temperature of 105 to 107 degrees. Fluids were forced to no effect, and a more hopeless case is seldom seen. Scarlet was applied just over the kidneys at a distance of eighteen inches for twenty minutes, all other areas covered. Two hours after, the child voided eight ounces of urine.

In some unusual and extreme cases that had not responded to other treatment, normal functioning has been restored by color therapy. At present, therefore, I do not feel justified in refusing any case without a trial. Even in cases where death is inevitable, much comfort may be secured.

There is no question that light and color are important therapeutic media, and that their adoption will be of advantage to both the profession and the people.

In the Woman's Hospital minutes of October 22, 1926 was this statement: "At a special meeting of the Board, Mrs. Kirk moved that Dr. Baldwin's resignation be accepted with regret. The motion was seconded and carried."

Finally, the minutes of January 27, 1927 recorded: "A letter from the Spectro-Chrome Therapists was read, deploring the action of the Woman's Hospital in requesting the resignation of Dr. Baldwin." A suggestion was made that Miss Bodine respond to the organization and enclose "Dr. Baldwin's appreciative letter to us and also stating that we had offered Dr. Baldwin a special department for her Spectro-Chrome work."

The AMA at that time was essentially controlled by one man, Dr. Morris Fishbein, who allegedly never practiced medicine and who graduated with a grade of 48 in Anatomy and never even spent the required two years as an intern.

Morris A. Bealle, editor of *Plain Talk Magazine*, published a book in 1945 titled *Medical Mussolini: A Comprehensive Text Book On Humanity's Scourge—Medical Politics*. Following are excerpts from the book which in no way reflect the AMA today since Dr. Fishbein was removed from his AMA affiliation in 1949:

The Medical Mussolini ... One of the briefest and most biting indictments of this closed shop feature of Morris Fishbein's AMA was delivered by the late beloved Dr. J. W. Hodge, M.D. of Niagara Falls, New York, who we presume must have been a prominent member of the Medical Dictator's first Black List:

The medical monopoly or medical trust, euphemistically called the American Medical Association, is not merely the meanest monopoly ever organized, but the most arrogant, dangerous and despotic organization which ever menaced a free people in this or any other age.

Any and all methods of healing the sick by means of safe, simple and natural remedies is sure to be assailed and denounced by the arrogant leaders of the AMA doctors' trust as 'fake, frauds, and humbugs'. Every practitioner of the healing art who does not ally himself with the medical trust is denounced a 'dangerous quack' and imposter by the predatory trust doctors.

Every sanitarian who attempts to restore the sick to a state of health by natural means without resort to the knife or poisonous drugs, disease imparting serums, deadly toxins or vaccines, is at once pounced up by these medical tyrants and fanatics, bitterly denounced, vilified and persecuted to the fullest extent.

Following the publication of the AMA article, the Woman's Hospital senior surgeon received a letter from a Dr. Beamis:

Dear Dr. Baldwin, In a reprint of an article published in the *Journal* of the American Medical Association, January 26, 1924, there appears the following statement: "*Spectro-Chrome* for March, 1923 contains an article on "Complicated Disorders Set Right by Spectro-Chrome" credited to Kate W. Baldwin, M.D., F.A.C.S., Senior Surgeon of the Woman's Hospital, Philadelphia."

According to this article, Susie T., age 9, who was admitted to the Woman's Hospital with a sloughed appendix and peritonitis, developed a pneumonia which was treated by Dr. Baldwin by Lemon, Turquoise and Magenta colored lights. Susie went home ... well, fat and happy.

Dinshah P. Ghadiali, using the title M.D., is the publisher of *Spectro-Chrome*. He is under house arrest in Buffalo charged with grand larceny for selling a course of lectures and leasing a colored light apparatus of alleged curative value for human ailments. We are wondering if the article in which your name is given is a correct statement. Our Society is somewhat interested in the outcome of this case, and we will very much appreciate your telling us if your name was used with authority.

Thanking you for the courtesy of an early reply, we are

Sincerely yours, Medical Society, County of Erie (Sd.) Louise W. Beamis, M.D., Secretary

Dr. Baldwin eagerly and immediately replied:

Dear Dr. Beamis, Your letter of June 9th is just received. The statement in the *Journal* of the American Medical Association of January 26th, 1924 is practically as written by me for the *Spectro-Chrome* magazine. Susie's was an emergency operation at nine o'clock at night. There was nothing left of the appendix to remove. There were quantities of pus. The wound could not be closed, free drainage was provided and the child put to bed with little hope that she would live until morning. For some days, an enema would simply pass through and out of the abdominal opening. Susie developed pneumonia. I did use Spectro-Chrome and eventually she did leave the hospital in good condition.

In the Woman's Hospital, I used Spectro-Chrome for many things to the satisfaction of the patients, the Staff and the Board. The results were approved by all interested until the article cited came out in the *Journal*. Then the Staff turned traitor. The Board appointed a Special Committee of five to investigate and a copy of its report I am enclosing. After this investigation, I was granted a large space for the work of Spectro-Chrome.

The American Medical Association continues to rate me as a fellow in good standing. Not the slightest effort to prove the truth has even been made by the A.M.A. or the Doctors. The simple fact that the A.M.A. made the statement against Spectro-Chrome was sufficient to condemn. At the time I wrote to the *Journal* stating facts. The courtesy of a reply was not granted. The letter was sent by registered mail and a return card showed that it was delivered. Eventually, this article was the cause of my losing my position on the Surgical Staff of the Woman's Hospital. The A.M.A. has not been just to one of its Members or to humanity; within the year of 1929 communications have been sent by the A.M.A. to several of my patients in the shape of a reprint of the article published in the 1924 *Journal* and a letter ridiculing Spectro-Chrome and me. Spectro-Chrome has more value as a therapeutic measure than all the Drugs and Serums manufactured. I would close my office tonight never to reopen, if I could not use Spectro-Chrome.

Respectfully,(Sd.) Kate W. Baldwin

What higher praise from a respected physician about a healing art could there be than "I would close my office tonight never to reopen, if I could not use Spectro-Chrome"? Still, the AMA was too powerful a force for her. For practicing a form of medicine whose results she swore by, Dr. Kate Baldwin, senior surgeon at Woman's Hospital, was removed from her position and became the first prominent victim of Dinshah's healing science.

The AMA consistently refused to investigate the healing science on which Dinshah spent many years of laborious research. Dinshah claimed that Spectro-Chrome met all the requirements of a complete scientific healing system based on unchangeable principles. Outside of purely surgical cases of a constructive or reparative nature, he said, Spectro-Chrome was applicable to all human ailments, with a precision not attainable by any other method known to science, and corroborated its results along mathematical, clinical, chromical and pathological lines. Dinshah asserted that many cases pronounced "beyond any human help" were successfully "normalated" by Spectro-Chrome: new skins were grown on large areas of a body burnt and completely destroyed by fire; born paralytics were made to walk; consumptives declared dying pulled out of bed in a few days and eventually restored to health; leaky hearts were rendered sound; arthritis and rheumatism were normalated after sufferers had been in agony for years; diabetes was removed and sufferers were given a new lease on life, without stopping the eating of starches and sugars;

cataracts stopped from further development; x-rays and radium destruction were fully repaired; certain types of blindness and deafness were removed; cancerous growth was controlled; it even helped alcoholics and drug addicts lose their craving for alcohol and drugs. All such near impossibilities, Dinshah maintained, were accomplished by Spectro-Chrome exclusively, using no drugs, manipulation or surgery, with no side effects whatsoever. Spectro-Chrome was not based on psychic or faith healing, since it worked equally well on infants and animals. Spectro-Chrome was a simple system that could be used by any individual in his or her home with scientific precision and accuracy. It was Dinshah's goal to have a Spectro-Chrome in every home.

The AMA repeatedly refused to accept Dinshah's challenge of investigating Spectro-Chrome, maintaining that the visible spectrum of light and color has no therapeutic effect and has absolutely no healing or curative value. If the AMA agreed to accept this challenge (preliminary results would take less than 90 days) and it proved effective, some followers of Spectro-Chrome contended it would have saved millions of people and their loved ones needless pain and suffering, in addition to saving billions of dollars spent on unnecessary drugs and surgery. They said that if Spectro-Chrome were to be offered as an auxiliary to existing medical science, it might possibly be acclaimed as the "most marvelous healing origination," since it would not affect the physician's livelihood.

Dinshah challenged the AMA to send seven representatives to take his course to investigate Spectro-Chrome, with first-class travel and hotel provided at no cost to the AMA, and if the AMA could prove that Spectro-Chrome made any false claims or that any of the thousands of case histories that were written up in his monthly magazine were untrue, or if Spectro-Chrome had no curative or healing value, then Dinshah, as he wrote in his letter to the medical organization, would present to the AMA all of his inventions, patents, copyrights, business and everything he owned, and give the

AMA an unconditional apology, and leave America and never return.

The AMA professed great skepticism about Spectro-Chrome, but to not even investigate it when scores of licensed physicians and other health professionals reportedly obtained successful results with it perhaps underscored a fear of it. If the general public were informed of Spectro-Chrome and subscribed to the lifestyle of Dinshah's philosophy behind his healing art, then people would rarely go to medical doctors, discontinue drinking liquor, quit smoking, and stop eating meat, and live without drugs and medicine as well as destructive surgery. People perhaps would live longer and much healthier lives. Sill, a number of selfless physicians were recommending their "incurable" patients to Specro-Chrome therapists, and these practitioners and patients reported getting near miraculous results.

8

DINSHAH FIRES BACK AT THE AMA

By the mid-1920s, Dinshah had trained people all over the U.S. on how to use Spectro-Chrome Therapy. These were not people "hypnotized" by his charisma or following a trend, nor were these ignorant people; among the Spectro-Chrome practitioners were surgeons, physicians, osteopaths, chiropractors, dentists, nurses, and other health professionals. There were also laypersons, and while it may be true that among them were some who may have felt desperate for a cure since conventional medicine could not help them, blind faith had to be eventually supplanted by some rational or scientific reasoning. To graduate from Dinshah's course and earn a diploma that entitled the graduate to use the initials "S.C.T." ("Spectro-Chrome Therapist") after his or her name required the person to pass an intensive course always given by Dinshah that rested, at least to one extent or another, on sound scientific principles.

Dinshah and many of his followers were not of any illusion that they would not be pilloried for using Spectro-Chrome and that the mere idea of Spectro-Chrome being a healing mechanism would not invite ridicule. After all, the idea that shining colored lights on the body could cure illnesses seemed, on the surface, absolutely absurd.

But science in its latest permutations showed that the impossible was possible — if there was science behind it. If, only a handful of years previous to Dinshah introducing Spectro-Chrome in 1920, anyone was told that music could be sent invisibly through the air to far-off places, that person would have thought the teller to be delusional. But it was around the same time that Dinshah introduced Spectro-Chrome that radio stations began broadcasting, sending waves of electrical energy through the air that a receiver in a home could recreate as audible music.

Quacks don't usually attract legions of health professionals who become lifetime users of the purveyor's methods and who consistently report successful results with the person's methods. They usually don't attract legions of health professionals who to one extent or another abandon their conventional medical or dental training and dedicate their practices to an unconventional form of medicine. But that is exactly what happened with Dinshah and his Spectro-Chrome Therapy shortly after it was introduced.

Dinshah and his followers — both health professionals and laypersons — expected to be challenged by conventional medicine — and the drug and other industries. They expected to hear stentorian chants and denunciations of "charlatan" and other similar derogatory names directed at them. Morris Fishbein, the AMA *Journal* editor, seemed bent on making his name by exposing quacks, and colored-light treatments for disease seemed a ripe candidate for his feverish mission.

In the wake of World War I there were efforts to ban various forms of German culture in the U.S., including instruction of the German language in schools. A teacher in the state of Nebraska, which prohibited using a foreign language as a means of instruction, was discovered teaching reading in German and fined. The decision was upheld by the Nebraska Supreme Court and the teacher appealed the decision to the U.S. Supreme Court. In a majority opinion Justice James Clark McReynolds wrote: "Mere knowledge of the German language cannot reasonably be regarded as harmful.

Heretofore it has been commonly looked upon as helpful and desirable. Plaintiff in error taught this language in school as part of his occupation. His right thus to teach and the right of parents to engage him so to instruct their children, we think, are within the liberty of the amendment."

Dinshah took the U.S. Supreme Court decision as due process of his right to practice unconventional medicine. Of it, he wrote in the April (Lemon) 1923 issue of *Spectro-Chrome*:

This is the very ideal I always have maintained and for which I have idolized the Constitution of the United States of America. The medical profession and the laws regulating the practice of "Medicine and Surgery" may be quite welcome and within their rights to choose, select and direct whatsoever laws their lobbied legislations may enact, but, as soon as they place their fingers on each and every Drugless Cult or System they are exceeding the birthrights of humanity, which are Liberty, Property, Security, and Contract. A person may be required to be licensed under certain laws to practice "Medicine and Surgery" but Drugless Cults and Systems of Healing are neither "Medicine nor Surgery" and the medical laws cannot touch them. Subsequently, the medical profession, in its horrible jealousy, got other laws passed through by pressuring legislations, terrorizing the various Drugless Practitioners and succeeding partially in placing their thumbs on the carotids of some weaklings. The underlying reasons of such partial success were the weaknesses in the public policies of such systems and the lax ways in which their teachings were conducted. The main feature of the fight hinged on the use of such Drugless Systems of the same textbooks on Anatomy, Physiology, Bacteriology, Histology, Pathology, Biology, Diagnoses and a number of other "lologies" as were taught in the regular medical schools and were "changed" every ten years to suit them. It was also owing to the followers of such Drugless Systems, appending the title of Dr. (Doctor, Driver or Debtor?) before their names, which irritated further the older school-members, perhaps deservedly.

When Spectro-Chrome Therapy was perfected and brought to the stage of commercial practical clinical application, the Originator had waded fully through these obstacles and legal complications. It was thought unwise to launch out, until this new Drugless Science could go before the whole medical and non-medical world and challenge boldly the right of the so-called Medical Profession to dictate to humanity what system should be used and how in order to alleviate the sufferings of the ailing. Step by step, in Spectro-Chrome Therapy, the Originator evolved a system, but which at one stroke swept clean the moth-eaten, ancient, valueless, destructive and inhuman doctrines foisted under the name of the healing art by ages of uncivilized and civilized so-called "sciences". In Spectro-Chrome Therapy, the Originator boiled down the known and to-the-general-public unknown knowledge of physical and metaphysical fundamentals, evolving a complete absolutely new science, art and profession, whose follower and practitioner can do everything the Drug or Drugless Systems aim at performing and at the same time whose knowledge did not need the usual Anatomy, Physiology, Histology, Pathology, Histology, Pathology, Biology, Bacteriology, and the intricate like. At one clean sweep, the Originator of Spectro-Chrome Therapy not only discarded the filthy, foul, dirty, obnoxious vaccines, serums, blood and urine therapies and the like, but, he threw into the scrap-heap of an ignorant past all the so-called methods of differential diagnosis of the various "strains" of human disorders, by which the ignorant public was hoodwinked into believing the regular Doctors as the "allwise".

The power of Spectro-Chrome Therapy in all these is so great that graduate after graduate is now discarding old views and bowing to the Divine Laws of Nature which are enunciated in Spectro-Chrome Therapy. They are now fast awakening to the fact that Spectro-Chrome Therapy needs no support of other systems to carve its way, in as much as it stands unrivalled on its own merits. It holds forth to the entire medical world the most potential challenge in the Healing Art and in as much as it follows entirely novel and universally unknown or unrecognized Laws of Nature, its followers and practitioners have positively nothing to fear in the existing manmade legislation governing other systems of healing.

Dinshah continued his censuring of the medical profession in the October (Purple) 1923 issue of *Spectro-Chrome*, where he trained his sight on the AMA. He wrote:

The duty of a journal is to be the upholder of the right, the defender of the down-trodden, the protector of the poor, the speaker of the unflinching truth, the enunciator of the most exact and precise facts.

For years, however, it has been an admitted matter that the American Medical Association as reflected in the conduct of its *Journal* has followed a line of apparently hoodwinking policy, endeavoring to be the angel in Heaven sitting on the throne of justice to adjudicate the merits of other systems of therapy from its own standpoint of knowledge and trying to represent to the world its great superiority by whipping the skin off those differing from its doctrines.

There was a time years ago, when, in the ignorance in which the public was submerged, it bowed in solemn reverence to the dictator who posed as the benefactor of the suffering sick. At that period, the persecution with which this abominable journalism that held its stick over leaders of other systems of therapy resulted on many untoward effects for those who were so unfortunate as not to gain the favor of this ugly monster. It therefor set up an oligarchy of tyranny by hogging the whole field of healing and through the assistance of stupid ignorant legislatures wove such a snare of oppression that the victims were glad to die at the bidding of this most un-American inhuman proposition.

The American Medical Association, in its past career, has established throughout the land a terrorizing Black Hand such as no commercial trust ever dared to dream. It is known and spoken of as the Medical Trust and by a cunning masterful affiliation with the Medical Examining Boards, Health Boards and all other so-called (Mahogany) boards it has created such a despotic administration, that even the boldest leaders of other therapies have avoided the uncanny contact of this gigantic trust as far as practicable.

This Medical Trust through its servile *Journal* has attacked and ruined the life work and reputation of many great researchers whose shoes it is not wise enough to clean. It has upheld only its own damnable poison therapy and destructive surgery and dashed the last hope of many a dying person who would otherwise have been saved by its obnoxious old-time "ethical" systems and persistent dogmatic interference. The M.D. has nothing but poisons and pills, potions and plasters, blisters, blasters and baboon glands, hog serums, dog serums, cow vaccines and pig pepsins, his utter dislike and inertia for progress has justly made him derided as "Doctor of Murder," "Doctor of Mules," "Mule Driver," "Money Dog," and now "Doctor of Monkey-glands" to give worn-out old debauchees the power lost by unnatural practices.

The *Journal* of the AMA is not recognized as an impartial reviewer, but has earned the demerit of a one-sided, partial one-eyed owl. Its single owl eye is blinded now by the dazzle of the science of Spectro-Chrome Therapy and the rising respect and confidence of the ailing public its followers are getting. It stands as it were dazed and blinded by the effulgence of the latest revelation in the healing art and in it sees the utter eventual destruction of the unholy temple of lie that the followers of poison therapy and master butchery have succeeded in creating throughout the length and breadth of the country.

This *Journal* of AMA in its foul public tactics bulldozed the Christian Scientists, Osteopaths, Electropaths, Chiropractors and others who dared differ from its unscientific attitude and now it has started similar tactics against the Originator of Spectro-Chrome Therapy, his system of healing and his positively graftless Spectro-Chrome Institute.

It published a long article deriding Dinshah and his qualifications, endeavoring also to besmirch the name of our most learned and estimable friend, Surgeon Kate W. Baldwin, M.D., F.A.C.S., S.C.T., whose name is blessed by hundreds who were saved from the surgical knife through her very skillful and timely use of Spectro-Chrome Therapy. It was this brave, progressive, courageous and masterful surgeon who saved Grace Shirlow from certain, sure and inevitable death when by her clothes catching fire her torso was nearly completely burnt and her skin was two-thirds destroyed. Let any M.D., any surgeon, look at the pictures in this article and judge for himself whether there *is* anything in *their* system or in *any other* system — drug or drugless — that could have saved the life of this pretty child.

This burned girl was taken to the Woman's Hospital in Philadelphia, Pennsylvania, where Dr. Kate W. Baldwin has been the Senior Surgeon for twenty years. When her long surgical experience plainly indicated to her that in the recognized methods of plastic surgery and skin grafting, dosing, dressing, doping and drugging, there was not a ghost of a chance for the injured girl to live through — her noble magnanimous heart throbbed to save the unfortunate patient through other means not as yet fully understood by the followers of so-called medical "science". Even at the risk of appearing unethical and unprofessional, this learned surgeon set aside all preconceived ideas, notions and methods and from the beginning started to treat Grace exclusively with Spectro-Chrome Therapy. There was no skin grafted, no surgical dressing used, no pill potion or powder administered, yet, the patient thrived and her bodily powers from within (as enunciated in Spectro-Chrome Therapy) built a new satin-like skin within a few months. Her kidneys, bowels, lungs and heart have functioned under Specto-Chrome Therapy most perfectly; even the temperature which went at times over 106 degrees Fahrenheit was controlled with the precision of a chronograph and brought down without delirium or any untoward symptoms.

This girl is now in the enjoyment of health and is a live monument to the labors of the Originator of Spectro-Chrome Therapy and the devotion, skill and accuracy of its pioneer followers.

And for such gracious and unselfish service to humanity, such dutiful use of her skill as a healer and such demonstration of her progressiveness as a capable and competent surgeon, this wonderful woman whose work was extolled as the most marvelous in the annals of surgery by eminent surgeons, got from the (un)American Medical Association through its obviously ignorant *Journal* editor nothing but ridicule and foolish derision. Such is the reward she as a Fellow of the AMA received from that disgraceful publication.

But that is not all — the end is not here; the end will come when Spectro-Chrome Therapy will put an end to this Octopus, whose disastrous practices none dared to speak about openly. That poor fish submerged in the ocean of crass ignorance, bloated into a stinking carcass of the most malodorous type because of its hoary antiquity has thought fit to attack the brain power, honesty and character of Dinshah, not knowing in what pouch it was inserting its grasping tentacles.

Whatever methods the leaders of other therapeutical systems may follow have nothing in common with Spectro-Chrome Therapy and the methods of its Originator. He abhors underhand tactics, crafty policies and grafty diplomacies. He prefers at all times to speak in the open without fear of consequences, where the weal of the suffering public demands that he speak.

It was here that Dinshah's letter of February 4, 1924 to the editor of the *Journal* of the American Medical Association was reproduced. It was sent by registered mail with receipt requested. The letter read:

On returning from my tour in California, my attention was drawn to an article published in your issue of January 26, 1924, under the heading "SPECTRO-CHROME THERAPY," attacking me personally as well as defaming my work and my Spectro-Chrome Institute.

My scientific and professional standing are so well known and recognized internationally during thirty-three years of a fearless and independent platform career that they need no vindication or justification; however, it appears that you never had the opportunity of investigating first-hand what Spectro-Chrome is and what it does.

As a humble servant of suffering humanity and injustice to yourself and the therapy you represent, I have the honor to invite you to appoint a committee of seven (7) of your representatives and send them to take my complete course on Spectro-Chrome Therapy with experiments and demonstrations at Hotel Manx, San Francisco, California, where my next class opens on Monday, the 24th of March 1924, at 7 p.m.

I hereby agree to pay all first class traveling and hotel expenses of your said seven (7) representatives and also to present the courses absolutely unconditional.

Furthermore, although I am known as a caustic speaker in denouncing the "Empiricism of Medical Science," I hereby pledge you my word of honor that not a word tending to derogate, discredit, disrespect, disrepute or dishonor your representative, their profession or their therapy will be uttered by me during the entire investigation and that they will be treated as my worthy and honored guests.

The above invitation stands good for two weeks from your receipt of this and your acceptance is requested within that period to enable me to remit in advance the stipulated expenses to your bankers and make other necessary arrangements.

Dinshah then continued to rail against the AMA in his *Spectro-Chrome* magazine article:

The above challenge which went by registered mail will remain as a permanent record against the cowardice, unfairness, pusillanimity and peanut-brained-ness of the most detestable organ of a cowardly trust which through covert means always endeavored to have the upper hand.

Ye Editor of the *Journal* of the AMA, you attacked my personality, integrity, character, unselfish work for humanity; I sent you a dignified request which, were you honest and integral, red-blooded and American, were you fair, just and clean-minded as well as competent, you would have either printed, answered, or accepted; but, in quietly ignoring my gentlemanly challenge you have proved forever your utter worthiness to wield the sacred editorial pen.

I challenge you and your entire Medical Trust. I defy you and your whole organization to show and prove a money-making scheme or a fraud on the public such as you have made me and my Spectro-Chrome Institute appear in your dastardly attack. I have said times without number on the platform during thirty-three years and now repeat emphatically that through me and my work your entire crack-brained edifice of drug therapy and destructive surgery will crumble to pieces and its bricks will be volatized into molecules, atoms, electrons, and beyond and blown off into where there is plenty of Sulphur and no winter!

Spectro-Chrome Therapy as taught by me is no fad imposition or fancy such as your fool article states. It has absolutely nothing in common with any other healing system and is not an improvement on the medical art. Medical "art" is too slimy to reform. While your whole medical science is nothing but stupid contradictions and empiricism, Spectro-Chrome is the very essence of the unknown hence unrecognized occult sciences of ages which its Originator researched and junctioned and presented to the world as its most humble servant.

... I ask for no quarters or mercy at your hands, ye Editor of the *Journal* of AMA! The owl's eye may be blinded by the glory of the Sun, but it is no fault of the Sun — it is the weakness of the owl's eye. You have started something — it will end not here but in the speedy disintegration of the fabric of the Medical Trust. Fight with all your might; I care not for you and your vicious tactics, for, at your hands I have nothing to fear.

Spectro-Chrome Therapy has come to stay and finally mark my words — within the next three years and less its power of Truth will throw the last monkey wrench in the cogs of your evil machinery and burst the entire engine of the repulsive Medical Trust never to recover its prior prestige or vaunted dignity and terrorizing influence.

For the *Journal* article which he found inaccurate, unfair, defamatory and appalling, Dinshah in turn disparaged and challenged the AMA. Would there be repercussions?

9

SPECTRO-CHROME CONVENTIONS

Dinshah remained undaunted by the forces he believed were out to quash Spectro-Chrome — what he called the "Medical Octopus". He had a cartoon that depicted this: an octopus with numerous tentacles labelled with the names of groups that used "underhanded, nefarious methods" but which Dinshah made "Squirm in agony". Among these groups were the American Medical Association, the American College of Surgeons, the National Better Business Bureau, boards of education, boards of pharmacy, the National Advertising Association, the Good Housekeeping Institute; also labelled in the tentacles were potions, pills, vaccines, serums, and dope; newspaper health columns; controlled radio; paid propaganda; and destructive surgery. The Medical Octopus swam in the Bay of Bunk on one side, and the Ocean of Ignorance on the other.

Though some people would criticize Dinshah for being a charlatan who made money by charging people to take his courses and selling Spectro-Chrome machines and equipment, he, in fact, used the relatively little money he made to support his family and feed back into his Spectro-Chrome Institute to fulfill its mission of bringing Spectro-Chrome to the public. Indeed, Spectro-Chrome courses were now given around the U.S.; there were state-wide Spectro-Chrome Therapist associations and there was an American Association of Spectro-Chrome Therapists. Dinshah, ever-tireless in trying to realize his dream of making Spectro-Chrome a mainstream healing system, delivered addresses at Spectro-Chrome graduation ceremonies, Spectro-Chrome state association meetings, and annual conventions of the American Association of Spectro-Chrome Therapists. He gave free public lectures in big cities and far-flung places, often attracting large crowds. He often traveled around with the bulky equipment necessary to demonstrate Spectro-Chrome Therapy. With programs and events and traveling arranged tightly he maintained schedules and itineraries just like a busy business executive. He sometimes traveled with his daughter, Kashmira, who was a Spectro-Chrome Therapist herself and an avid writer for the healing system's monthly magazine. Kashmira often wrote colorful chronicles of their train trips through small towns, large cities, deserts, forests and wilderness, over hills, alongside rivers and around canyons, in all regions of the country.

As he traveled the country Dinshah invited members of the press to attend his lectures and investigate his science. Typical of this sincere solicitation was the following letter Dinshah wrote on May 5, 1924 from the Hotel Gowman in Seattle, Washington to the editor of the *Daily Journal of Commerce*, the largest commercial newspaper in the northwest:

As advertised in your newspaper you will please note that I am here on my visit to place before the public my original system of treatment of dis-eases by Attuned Color Waves, which entirely discards all drugs and destructive surgery.

My work has been presented during the last four years from the Atlantic to the Pacific Coast and as usual has created antagonism from the orthodox American Medical Association, in which, most singularly, Henry Ford's newspaper, *The Dearborn Independent*, also recently joined.

Enclosed you will find true copies of the opposition and my answers.

I am here to present my work to independent, impartial American judgment and as the public naturally looks to you for guidance, it will be appreciated if during my presence here you will send your duly accredited representative to take my complete course at my expense.

This offer is unconditional, places you under no obligation whatever and is made solely with the intention of giving you the honest opportunity to secure unprejudiced, full information from the original source.

The assistant editor of the newspaper, M. W. Bean, responded in a letter dated May 12, 1924, that a representative of the paper, E. M. Desmond, "has been appointed to investigate the work you are carrying out in Seattle."

E. M. Desmond attended the course and delivered the following unsolicited testimony on the last night:

A few words of appreciation to Colonel Dinshah P. Ghadiali, president of Spectro-Chrome Institute:

Today, being the closing day of the Spectro-Chrome Therapy class, I feel it my duty to write, even if briefly, my candid opinion of Colonel Dinshah and his work.

I am not obliged to do and was told by him that should I write anything, to write what I really believed. If I believe his work is a fraud, his motives mercenary only, or if he is what he represents himself to be — a learned man, a teacher and a benefactor to suffering humanity — "to write without restriction."

I cannot express myself with sufficient emphasis in a few words, but know that a long message sometimes loses its value and appears flowery and exaggerated.

Previous to the opening of the Seattle class in Spectro-Chrome Therapy, I had the pleasure of meeting the man. I was immediately impressed with his forceful personality, sincerity and the good work he is doing. He told me then that he had a standing offer to the newspapers in each city he visits to send a representative to investigate his work without any expense to the newspaper or the representative selected. His offer was unconditional and without any obligation whatever.

I asked permission of the *Daily Journal of Commerce* to allow me to take advantage of the offer. It was granted and I took the full course.

If I had paid personally a thousand dollars for this course, I would thank Colonel Dinshah for the good it did me, finding myself now a far better man in every way — physically and mentally. I am indeed grateful to him for this exceptional opportunity.

The Seattle class started May 12th ending tonight, May 27th, consisting ordinarily of twenty-four discourses in twelve nights — two each night. Colonel Dinshah voluntarily stayed over two extra nights at a financial loss to complete this Seattle work in a satisfactory manner. The class consisted of forty-six students, men and women of stability and intelligence, physicians, surgeons, osteopaths, sanipractors, chiropractors and people in other walks of life. Attendance at every discourse was 100 per cent.

Sitting among these people I never once heard a word of disappointment or reproach, which was evidenced by the offer of Colonel Dinshah to refund the enrollment fee of One Hundred Dollars to anyone disappointed or dissatisfied. No one came forward or as much uttered a word of complaint.

It is my absolute belief that Colonel DInshah is an honorable man, "practises what he preaches," and that he is doing a great good as a teacher and benefactor to humanity, suffering or otherwise.

Like all inventors and pioneers in new fields he has an uphill fight and is being attacked by certain powerful interests — some through ignorance of the man and his motives, others through their nature to attack anyone who does not accept their obsolete ideas.

In conclusion, I can truthfully state that I believe in Colonel Dinshah, the good he is doing, and Spectro-Chrome Institute.

This is my finding as an investigator and as a newspaperman acting as accredited representative for the *Daily Journal of Commerce*. Spectro-Chrome Institute has my full permission to use it as seems fit.

When Mr. Desmond concluded his remarks the entire class gave a robust round of applause.

Annual conventions of the American Association of Spectro-Chrome Therapists were exciting events packed with speeches and health professionals and laypersons reporting on the successful results they obtained with Spectro-Chrome Therapy. The Third Annual Convention held at the Institute's headquarters at 2401 North Broad Street in Philadelphia brought in a large number of people from all over the country as well as representatives of several newspapers. Among the Spectro-Chrome graduates who reported successful results with the therapy at the convention were Kate W. Baldwin, M.D.; Martha J. Peebles, M.D.; Sydney Smith, M.D.; Welcome A. Manor, M.D.; Charles Grapek, M.D.; Charles Rosendale, M.D.; Alice Norton, D.D.S.; Samuel Grants, D.D.S.; John A. Callahan, D.O.; Alice Gants, D.O.; Paul Koenig, D.C.; Bert C. Smith, D.C.; and numerous layperson practitioners. Dinshah himself delivered an address and gave a demonstration of a new invention of his called a "sympathometer" (a special clock used to indicate times to tonate). Annual conventions usually took place over a few days. Attendees would be invited, if the conventions took place in the Philadelphia area, to visit the Spectro-Chrome Institute in Malaga, where, after debarking from "automotive omnibuses" provided to them, they would go to the Central Office and Research Laboratory in the main building and from the Reception Room would tour the President's Office, Secretarial Office, Slide Room,

Bulb Room, the Experimental Research Room, the High Tension Electricity Room, the Static Machine Room, the Projection Room, the Stock Room, and Dinshah's bedroom, which he described in his magazine as "a bare floor with one ordinary bed, one folding chair and one plain dresser with a small writing table (worth in all less than fifty dollars)." The tour included other facilities away from the main building such as the Engine Room, the garage for the Institute's vehicles, and the grounds of the estate.

Medals were sometimes bestowed upon Spectro-Chrome Therapists at the annual conventions. For instance, at the Fourth Annual Convention a silver medal was awarded to Emma H. Gabriel, N.D. [Naturopathic Doctor or Doctor of Naturopathy], S.C.T., for her work on a three-year-ten-month-old child named Anna Schoener. Anna could not walk and she could only stand when held by both arms. She had been taken to several Philadelphia hospitals and her father, a city police officer, was told that there was nothing that could be done to help the child. She would never walk. One hospital advised minor operations with the girl to wear braces but could not guarantee these procedures would work. The father consented only to the braces but even with them the girl could not stand on her feet by herself.

On May 23, 1924, the girl's father brought her to Spectro-Chrome Therapist Emma Gabriel. Gabriel began by using lemon systemic (full body). The father remained with the girl in the darkened room and shouted out for Gabriel, whom he told the girl was able to stretch out, something she had never done before. Still, the girl was unable to turn herself.

Four systemic lemon treatments were followed by yellow, orange and red treatments. Then the girl got measles and the chicken pox and had home treatments. When she got better she returned to Gabriel's office and was given systemic green and lemon treatments. The child was taken off meat, which she liked, and was placed on a vegetarian diet. White bread was eliminated from her diet and she was given whole wheat for breakfast. Treatments were continued, which the child found difficult as it was hard for her to lay still in the dark for an extended period of time, and she often slept in the course of the sessions.

Gabriel went away for the first half of September and upon return inquired about the Anna's health. The child had dysentery and then the grippe, for which she received medical help. Her father could not bring her in for Spectro-Chrome treatments because his tours of duty had changed. But on October 7, 1924, he began to bring her in again. Anna could now walk while using one hand to hold on to a table or some other object. Gabriel then treated the girl three times a week administering mostly yellow and orange treatments. Soon, the girl could stand by herself as she counted to ten.

Gabriel was so pleased with the results that she brought young Anna to a convention of the American Association of Spectro-Chrome Therapists. As she wrote in *Spectro-Chrome* magazine about Anna's progress:

> She is able to go up and down the stairs alone. In good weather, I have her three sisters take her walking on the street. She still tires very easily. She walks very carefully, but there is now full control over the legs and there is perfect coordination. The muscles of her legs are soft and pliable. She gained over ten pounds since last May and grew four inches. The child seems to be happy; she laughs and talks all the time while under treatment. A few days ago, she called me and said "Can't you hurry up this 'light'?" I hope to report this case in the near future as being altogether righted.

Gabriel did indeed follow up with a report in the October (Purple) 1925 issue of the magazine. She wrote:

> The readers of *Spectro-Chrome* will remember the girl Anna Schoener whom I had last year before the Annual Convention of Spectro-Chrome Therapists. The little tot now walks alone. During the early Spring and the beginning of Summer, I was quite

discouraged as the child made so little progress, but that was main due to interrupted treatment. There seemed to be nobody at home who could bring the youngster to the office. During the Summer months and the vacation time, her older sister brought her regularly twice a week and now we have our reward.

When I came back from my vacation, her sister brought her down again and behold!! — Anna came in walking alone!! For a moment, I held my breath when I saw her. She is a little unsteady as yet; she walks more on her toes; the heels won't come down as yet, but I am sure in a little while she will be alright. I see a difference in her every week. Her treatment is always Orange systemic for an hour. The last time her father (a policeman) brought her, he took both my hands and said "Doctor, it is accomplished! Let me know in time when the next Convention is; I have to have a leave of absence for that day to bring Anna to the convention myself."

Anna's father took her to the Fifth Annual Convention held on December 27, 1925. Anna was able to walk there, but with her father's assistance. But less than two years later, with Spectro-Chrome treatments, Anna was able to walk to school on her own. At the Seventh Annual Convention held on November 28, 1927 at the Hotel Lorraine in Philadelphia, Dr. Emma Gabriel asked Anna to walk across the Convention Hall which she did without anyone helping her.

10

TROUBLE FOR DINSHAH:
REPERCUSSIONS?

After the AMA *Journal* article was published and Dr. Kate Baldwin was effectively terminated from her position at Women's Hospital in Philadelphia, other Spectro-Chrome Therapists started feeling the heat of the medical octopus pressure cooker in practicing the healing science. In Atlanta, a medical doctor-Spectro-Chrome Therapist was threatened with expulsion by the County Medical Society because he had a layperson Spectro-Chrome Therapist working with him. The Medical Society ordered the physician not to use Spectro-Chrome Therapy unless the group officially approved it. In the same city Cleo V. Butner, whose Spectro-Chrome practice was assailed by the County Medical Society was nevertheless charged a $150 license fee to be a practitioner; she felt that the fee was levied since Spectro-Chrome Therapists cut into medical doctors' income and that the medical profession manipulated the licensing authorities.

There were reports of many other Spectro-Chrome Therapists running into trouble but the biggest trouble came to Dinshah himself. In April 1925 he traveled the Pacific Coast to bring Spectro-Chrome to audiences in the American far West. But rather than being a journey of edification it turned out to be a plunge into an abyss of distress. He was maligned by various organizations there, vicious lies were spread about him and his wife and daughter, and his life was even threatened. But most despairingly, he was charged with violating a U.S. federal law, the Mann Act, also referred to as the White Slave Traffic Act.

Dinshah traveled with a female secretary and he was accused of transporting the young lady across state lines for immoral purposes. His alleged offense was a felony, subject to imprisonment and a fine.

A trial was held in the United States District Court in Portland, Oregon. During the trial the girl stated she had been placed in a hypnotic trance for ten months. Because Dinshah was a Hindu, she said, he had magical powers, although no supporting evidence was introduced. The trial lasted 14 days and on December 4, 1925, Dinshah, who for the first time retained attorneys to represent him in a trial, was convicted of violating the Mann White Slave Act. He adamantly denied the charges and declared he had no supernatural powers, no mystical powers, no capabilities of inducing trances in others, and pleaded not guilty in the courtroom presided over by Judge Robert S. Bean. But it was all to no avail and Dinshah believed that he had been framed — that the medical profession and the Ku Klux Klan were behind the travesty of his trial. Nevertheless, his plea of innocence and his conjectures of nefarious powers behind the alleged trumped-up charges couldn't absolve him of guilt in the court's eyes and so, at the age of 52, he was sentenced to five years at the McNeil Island penitentiary in Washington state and a fine of $5,000.

Dinshah appealed the verdict to the California Circuit Court of Appeals which to his chagrin upheld the verdict that he used mesmerism to put the girl in a hypnotic trance. So livid was Dinshah about the events that led to his being found guilty that he wrote a two-volume book about what he asserted was a frame-up called *Railroading a Citizen* that was published on May 27, 1926.

Dinshah took his case to the U.S. Department of Justice and John Garibaldi Sargent, the U.S. attorney general. He brought a writ of certiorari to the U.S. Supreme Court, which denied it. He went to the Pardon Attorney of the United States, James A. Finch, who, upon receiving 65 affidavits pertaining to the case from Dinshah, conducted an investigation. Finch subsequently requested Calvin Coolidge, the president of the U.S., to grant Dinshah a 60-day respite. Then, while he was on vacation in North Dakota, Coolidge granted Dinshah another respite of 30 days. Dinshah was hopeful he would not serve time but Attorney General Sargent wired him that pursuant to government rules that in order for a president to grant a pardon a person must actually be a prisoner in order to be pardoned.

Dinshah requested the Pardon Attorney to transfer his incarceration to the United States penitentiary at Atlanta, Georgia, and a Commitment Order was signed. He was ordered to voluntarily surrender to the U.S. Marshal in Atlanta on or before June 10, 1927. During his respites he continued his personal mission to alleviate human suffering by treating the sick and he pressed on with his business with his Spectro-Chrome Institute and the American Association of Spectro-Chrome Therapists. There was also a practical matter: the institute had a $5,000 loan out and the bank was closing in (a personal loan from a friend would eventually stop the banks from taking the deed to the property).

Dinshah's application for executive clemency went to George Farnum, the Assistant Attorney General, and he waited anxiously for a reply. There was no immediate response, and on the afternoon of Saturday, September 10, 1927 two U.S. Marshals came to Dinshah's Malaga, New Jersey office with a warrant charging him as a "fugitive from justice". The marshals whisked him off to the Mercer County Jail in Trenton, New Jersey; three days later, Dinshah P. Ghadiali, the scientist with many honorary degrees whose healing art numerous medical professionals swore by, went off to the federal penitentiary in Atlanta.

At the Atlanta facility, the largest federal penitentiary in the U.S., every detail of the prisoners' personal lives was scrutinized: medical examinations, letters they sent out, letters mailed to them, and people who came to see them. While serving time at the Atlanta penitentiary an uprising was brewing that Dinshah helped squash by supplying information to authorities there at the risk of his own life, and he also bravely exposed corruption at the facility. The U.S. Senate ordered the Department of Justice to investigate what happened at the Atlanta penitentiary. By that time Dinshah had already served thirteen months of his sentence and he requested a pardon. To his dismay, the Parole Board wouldn't grant the parole but cut down his sentence to three years.

The Parole Board consisted of the prison warden, the prison superintendent and the facility's physician, and they refused to release Dinshah. They expressed their gratitude for his service to the prison by sequestering him in a steel cage eighteen inches below the ceiling. His family sent him food packages as he was not given vegetarian meals but the same food as others. He gave his unacceptable meal portions to his fellow inmates and on Wednesdays they repaid him by loading him with all their mashed potatoes.

For part of the time he served at the Atlanta penitentiary Dinshah shared a cell with a vicious murderer and a notorious counterfeiter. Of this setup, he said, "A prison is a school of crime. I entered it as an honest man, but from constant conversation of prisoners I could not help but acquire knowledge of how to be a first-class lock-picker, safe-cracker and forger, had I wished to pursue such trades in later life."

Being an outspoken man he rapped the prison system, which, as he witnessed first-hand, threw white-collar convicts together with hardened criminals. Dinshah was locked up for much of the time in a basement stall formerly occupied by government horses.

Rampant corruption existed in the Atlanta penitentiary and Dinshah managed to expose this to U.S. Department of Justice officials. Thomas C. Wilcox of the Department of Justice and a close associate of the U.S. president clandestinely sent a letter to Dinshah in prison that appointed him a special agent of the U.S. government. Dinshah quickly destroyed the letter so the plan could not be exposed. Almost five months later, on February 18, 1929, Dinshah received a commutation, effective immediately, from President Calvin Coolidge. After 17-and-a-half months of time served, Dinshah was released from the Atlanta penitentiary.

The release couldn't have come at a better time for Dinshah, who was as determined as ever to bring his healing system to the masses. He would now be able to attend the Eighth Annual Convention of the American Association of Spectro-Chrome Therapists to be held in the auditorium of the Spectro-Chrome Institute in Malaga on Saturday, March 30, 1929 (postponed at his request from November 28, 1928 because he expected to be released from prison), and there were other upcoming Spectro-Chrome conventions after that. After what he considered was an unjust incarceration that tied up his life for more than a year-and-a-half, Dinshah could get back to the work he lived for, because he was finally unfettered from legal persecution. At least for the moment.

11

DINSHAH LOOKS OUT FOR
SPECTRO-CHROME PRACTITIONERS

Dinshah was concerned that legal authorities would continue to not just pursue him, but Spectro-Chrome practitioners everywhere, and he felt compelled to protect his graduates. Spectro-Chrome annual conventions became important forums not just for practitioners to tell about the success of their cases and share therapeutic information but for Dinshah to discuss means to avoid legal persecution.

For example, at the Ninth Annual Convention, which was actually a joint convention of the Scientific Order of Spectro-Chrome Metrists and the American Association of Spectro-Chrome Therapists held on November 28, 29 and 30, 1929 at the auditorium of the Spectro-Chrome Institute in Malaga, New Jersey, Dinshah pledged to do his best to safeguard Spectro-Chrome graduates "from the tactics of the medical trust". Trying to disassociate Spectro-Chrome from conventional medicine, and thereby the legal constraints that may make practitioners liable for practicing medicine without a license, he said that:

> Spectro-Chrome had nothing common with any system of healing, much less medicine and the laws governing the practice of

medicine had nothing to do with Spectro-Chrome, which was the science of automatic precision having no diagnosis, no drugs, no manipulation, no surgery. The medical laws were all one-sided and arbitrary. They were worded most cunningly to keep out and bar every conceivable system of healing, acting thus as a monopoly of the most pernicious character.

Dinshah had by now stopped the selling and leasing of Spectro-Chrome equipment to keep unauthorized and dishonest people from using it and marring the reputation of trained practitioners. He also wanted "to protect the public from fraud and misrepresentation" as federal laws did "not allow an equipment to be regulated or restricted in regard to its use." It wasn't just fake machines that were being peddled, but fake color slides as well. "It were better for Spectro-Chrome Institute to lose its income at present," he said, "than to prosper on the quackery of unauthorized practitioners and lose its reputation for service to mankind." This was a big financial sacrifice for Dinshah, as equipment sales were a vital source of revenue to keep his institute running. Around this time Dinshah also substituted the word "Metry" for "Therapy" in the Spectro-Chrome nomenclature since the system, with many new devices he invented to make diagnosis easier for practitioners, "was now one of measurement and not only for healing."

In the first day afternoon session of the Ninth Annual Convention Dinshah announced that the Scientific Order of Spectro-Chrome Metrists had formed into a corporation and that it had several purposes, among them:

to advance, demonstrate and practice Spectro-Chrome Metry, the science of automatic precision for the measurement and restoration of the human radio-active and radio-emanative equilibrium by attuned color waves as originated and taught by Dinshah P. Ghadiali, exclusively and without the use of any auxiliary science...to establish an international nucleus for the exchange of views among Spectro-Chrome Metrists, Graduates of Spectro-Chrome Institute ... to organize and maintain bureaus of training in Spectro-Chrome Metry for enlightenment through discourses, publication and similar means of literary and scientific dissemination ... to encourage such sensible legislation as will promote the cause of Spectro-Chrome Metry...to extend by Spectro-Chrome Metry, aid and relief to those who seek and merit it ... to spread Spectro-Chrome Metry throughout the world.

By the 1930s there were Spectro-Chrome groups all around the U.S. They were called "Planets" and they were run by authorized Spectro-Chrome users who were certified as "normalators". They would treat, or "tonate", ill people and had periodic meetings in which they would report on their cases. Their reports cited numerous successful treatments and the users were generally very optimistic about the healing science they practiced but they were quite aware of what they — and Dinshah — were up against.

Dinshah laid out strict rules for Planet groups, as he would write in *Spectro-Chrome*:

Our affairs are strictly for Spectro-Chrome education and not for clubbing as a gossip house ... Sufferer Chart must be in the hands of the Chairman, for proper discussion. Refrain from haphazard advice ... Spectro-Chrome Technique must be properly followed. None, whether graduate or Provisional Member has authority to alter it or use it "as they please". Spectro-Chrome is *not* medicine to be left to the individual opinion or mental reservation of the user. The Science is built on precise mathematics and cannot be subjected to the mental caprices and whims of any person. Therefore, an Affiliate not following the Rules is creating Violation of our Constitution and if duly charged and on Investigation proved "guilty" is liable to discipline.

And there were more warnings. Dinshah was rigidly strict in

having the Institute's rules followed and noted that many people had been expelled for violations, and that he would have "no hesitation in expelling a whole group".

For a Planet to form there had to be a minimum of five graduates of the Spectro-Chrome Institute who were in good standing with the Institute. Because there could be more than one Planet in a city, each Planet had in its name the number of its order of establishment, for example, First Detroit Michigan Planet. Each Planet had three officers: a deputy, sub-deputy, and a recorder.

Named after the cities and states of their locations, there were Planets in several places around the U.S.: St. Louis, Missouri; Milwaukee, Wisconsin; Wilmington, Delaware; Detroit, Michigan; Cleveland, Ohio; Chicago, Illinois; Allentown, Pennsylvania; Portland, Oregon; New York, New York. Planets met monthly and the meetings were open to all Spectro-Chrome Affiliates (an Affiliation card had to be presented). At the meetings, information on the Spectro-Chrome science was dispensed and affiliates had the opportunity to speak about their cases. Recorders typed transcripts of the meetings and sent them to the Spectro-Chrome Institute for publication in *Spectro-Chrome* magazine, but beginning in the 1930s the last names of affiliates were often left out so they could not be hounded by legal authorities.

12

THE GRAND LARCENY TRIAL

On March 7, 1930 Dinshah drove into Buffalo, New York to give a class on Spectro-Chrome. The temperature was 39 degrees Fahrenheit in this upstate New York town, infamous for its frigid temperatures and snowy winters. By this time, Dinshah had already given 54 classes around the U.S., most on the east and west coasts, but also in some large cities between the coasts like Chicago, Detroit and Cleveland. Although Spectro-Chrome practitioners continued to run into trouble with the law and Dinshah had served time in federal prison after being found guilty on charges unrelated to Spectro-Chrome, his healing art continued to be widely practiced and receive national media attention.

Upon his arrival in Buffalo, Dinshah sent circulars advertising his free public lectures to the *Buffalo Courier-Express* and the *Buffalo Times*. The *Courier-Express* printed the ad in its March 10, 1930 issue but the *Times* refused. Dinshah went to see the editor, G. B. Parker, with his bulky apparatus that he had brought with him and even after he had explained and demonstrated his work Parker still rebuffed him.

Dinshah began his 55th Spectro-Chrome class in Buffalo on

Monday, March 17, 1930. There were 14 new students enrolled and three people who had previously trained with Dinshah. The newcomers included Dr. Oscar Keener, President of the Buffalo Optometric Society, from Kenmore, New York, and Bertha McNamara, a nurse. One of the repeaters was Welcome A. Manor, M.D. Houseman Hughes of Buffalo was also among the students. The class concluded on March 31 and so much interest was aroused that Dinshah was asked to give another course.

So gratified was the class that had just concluded that on March 31, 1930 the students delivered the following letter to Dinshah:

Dear Sir, We, the undersigned, members of the 55th class in Spectro-Chrome Metry, wish to extend to you our sincere thanks and appreciation for having given us this opportunity to grasp some of the wonders of nature. The 30 discourses presented alone have an education value that is fully worth the charge made for it. Your knowledge of science and the demonstrations made were very amazing and cannot help but create in any person's mind the thought of how it is possible for anyone to master all you have accomplished in one lifetime.

Your methods of teaching in carrying the course through step by step unfolds a world of knowledge that is invaluable, and is brought to the student in such a manner that enables anyone with a limited education to grasp the fundamentals very readily. We do not know of any other course where such valuable information could be obtained in such a short period, and it is our feeling we have been well repaid for the sacrifices made in devoting our time here for the past fifteen days.

With the success of the 55th class, Dinshah commenced another, and on its last day, on Monday, May 12, 1930, he was approached by two plainclothes men who said that they were acting on a complaint by one of his former students, Houseman Hughes, who asserted that he had been bilked out of $200. Dinshah accompanied the officers to the police headquarters, where Commissioner Austin J. Roche conducted an inquiry. Hughes was also present. Commissioner Roche asked the complainant some questions, to which Hughes gave some evasive replies.

"How is it that you signed and swore before a notary public a Contract for Hire of a Graduate Model Spectro-Chrome Equipment with a $200 refundable deposit?" the Commissioner asked.

Hughes quickly responded that Dinshah had "hypnotized" the class.

After hearing Dinshah's side of the story, the Police Commissioner released him. Dinshah promptly returned to his class at the Lafayette Hotel and after completing the lesson dismissed the students at 1 a.m.

In early June, Dinshah had just arrived in Rochester when he received an urgent phone call from Dr. Keener. The optometrist informed Dinshah that there was a warrant out for his arrest.

Houseman Hughes, a man who admitted that he had been declared "insane" by three doctors seemed unusually persistent in his efforts to have Dinshah incarcerated. When detectives arrived at Dinshah's hotel suite the Parsee Indian was dressed and waiting for them, much to their surprise. They served him with a warrant for grand larceny and Dinshah surrendered. He left his luggage with the hotel clerk and was taken to the police headquarters where he spent the night in jail.

Dinshah paced the floor until the next morning. After refusing to eat breakfast, he was fingerprinted and photographed. Some of the officers poked fun at Dinshah and called him "Ghandi". Two detectives from the Buffalo Police Department picked up Dinshah at three a.m. and they drove 70 miles to the city's police headquarters. During this trip, Dinshah spoke of his science and one of the arresting officers expressed interest in it. Dinshah later sent literature on Spectro-Chrome to his home.

At the police station Dr. Welcome A. Manor and William S. Harrison, a realtor and former student of Dinshah's, arranged bail and had him released. They also told Dinshah of the nature of his arrest. After Police Commissioner Roche had dismissed Houseman's complaint against him the mechanic had attempted to have him arrested but learned that Dinshah had already checked out of the hotel where he was staying. He had then gone to the district attorney's office. Without any investigation the case was taken to the grand jury and based solely on Hughes' testimony an indictment was rendered. Hughes, along with Bertha McNamara who would appear as a witness for the prosecution, had signed the March 31, 1930 testimonial of the 55th class of Spectro-Chrome.

After much postponing, the trial finally began on Tuesday, April 28, 1931 in the Erie County Court. Dinshah was accused of:

> "Grand Larceny second degree, contrary to the Penal Laws, Section 1290, 1296, in that he the said Dinshah P. Ghadiali on the 29th day of March 1930, at the city of Buffalo in this county did feloniously steal $175 from Houseman Hughes by falsely representing and pretending that a certain instrument and machine could cure any and all human disease and ailments and that the glass in the said machine and instrument was specially prepared and contained certain lines and scripts, whereas in truth and in fact the said machine and instrument could not cure all human disease and ailments and the said glass in the said machine was not specially prepared and did not contain the said lines and scripts."

The indictment was issued without any research having been performed on Dinshah's healing science. Dinshah wrote that the reference to the "lines and scripts" was "a pack of humor".

On the day of the trial, sitting on the Supreme Court bench was Justice Thomas H. Noonan. The courtroom was packed with users of Spectro-Chrome, students who took Dinshah's Spectro-Chrome course, attorneys who worked in the area, curious spectators, as well as newspaper reporters.

Indeed, the trial received much media attention. The *Rochester American* referred to Dinshah as a "mystic" and mentioned in its article that Dinshah had been imprisoned in 1925 in violation of the Mann Act. The Rochester *Democrat and Chronicle* and newspapers in Buffalo also covered the case.

The key issue at the trial was whether Dinshah's machine was able to do what he claimed it could. Dinshah had no legal representation, as he preferred to defend himself. Twelve men sat on the jury including salesmen, a baker, a farmer, a clerk, and a milkman. When Dinshah's secretary whispered to him her concern about these laypersons not being able to comprehend his science, he said that they would in fact be good jurors, and proceeded to tell her how their work would enable them to comprehend various scientific aspects, or, in the case of the salesmen, how their backgrounds would enable them to see through the claims of Housman Hughes with regard to the Contract for Hire that he had signed.

In his opening remarks to the jury, the assistant district attorney, Leo J. Hagerty, essentially said:

> Housman Hughes took the course for $150. What was his object in paying it? He was told Spectro-Chrome cured all diseases — that defendant Dinshah P. Ghadiali, with numerous titles, told him it was foolish to go for operations. The machine is patented. The defendant is a magician who knows only how to make those colored glasses — they are special, with healing qualities, but I say that they are nothing but window glasses — five cents a glass.

ADA Hagerty called Houseman Hughes to the stand as the people of New York State's first witness. After taking him through the whole chronology of how he was allegedly duped by Dinshah, he asked: "Did he say anything about this Spectro-Chrome or these colored glasses being able to cure any and all diseases and ailments?"

"Everything but broken bones," Hughes responded.

A battery of witnesses for the prosecution claiming Dinshah's machine did not do what he claimed it could do were then direct-examined by the ADA and cross-examined by Dinshah, who tried to poke holes in their accounts. At the end of the day, the newspapers ridiculed Dinshah.

On the second day of the trial the ADA called to the stand Melvin C. Reinhart, a physicist, who was employed by the New York State Institute for the Study of Malignant Diseases, also known as the Gratwick Laboratories. He said Hughes had come to him and at his request he had

> made a spectrographic test, not only of the glass in the case here, but of the entire optical system and of the light source of the apparatus, both the ultraviolet spectrographic test and a visible spectrographic test.

After several questions the ADA asked:

> Then your examination of all the glass in the machine, including the colored glass and the other glasses which were shown to you, convinced you that this glass is nothing more than ordinary glass which can be duplicated by any standard manufacturer?

"Yes," Reinhart answered.

Then Dinshah grilled him, leading to a long exchange of scientific jousting that was sometimes contentious, and which seemed to entertain all those in the courtroom. Throughout, Reinhart denied having any knowledge of the effect of color on the human body.

The justice ordered a brief recess after which ADA Hagerty brought onto the stand another prosecution witness, Earl L. Eaton, a licensed physician in New York State. Eaton stated that he did not think an apparatus such as Dinshah's machine would have any value as a therapeutic agent.

After this, the first witness for the defense was called, a medical doctor named Welcome Anson Hanor from Silver Creek, New York, with offices in Dunkirk and Buffalo, New York. On the stand, Hanor said he had met Dinshah when they were both vice-presidents of the Allied Medical Association and that he had taken Dinshah's course in Spectro-Chrome Metry when it was offered in Bradford, Pennsylvania.

Dinshah: Kindly look at that equipment behind you. After your graduation, did you get an equipment like that?

Hanor: I did.

Dinshah: Did you use it?

Hanor: I did.

Dinshah: In what work did you use that equipment?

Hanor: I used it in connection with my practice and general cases as they presented, that I thought might be indicated. I used I it in burns, I used in in arthritis, diabetes, cancer, empyema, pulmonary tuberculosis, enlarged tonsils.

Dinshah: Did you use it in any cases of dementia praecox or insanity?

Hanor: Yes, sir.

Dinshah: Any heart diseases?

Hanor: I have.

Dinshah: Any intestinal disorders?

Hanor: Constipation.

Dinshah: Did you use it for any cases of low blood pressure?

Hanor: I have.

Dinshah: What were the results from your own medical standpoint with the use of that equipment?

Hanor: They were excellent.

Dinshah: Did you get any cases rejected according to the old doctrine of medicine?

Hanor: If I accepted cases that have been rejected? I have.

Dinshah: As incurable, so called?

Hanor: Well, I have had cases that were getting worse. I don't know that the physicians refused to treat them.

Justice: Whether they declared them hopeless, you don't know that?

Hanor: Well, I think I do, if I can have a little time to think. I have treated so many cases.

Dinshah: I shall put another question, doctor.

Hanor: I am treating one at present, that has been pronounced hopeless.

Dinshah: What case is that?

Hanor: That I have not dismissed, but the patient is improving.

Dinshah: What case is it?

Hanor: Case of cancer.

Dinshah: Where?

Hanor: Syracuse, New York, diagnosed by the x-ray as having cancer and pronounced hopeless. They have called me in to give her what relief I might be able to expecting nothing more and with that understanding. The patient has become active and is getting around the streets and so far as I can ...

Dinshah: Is improving?

Hanor: The ultimate outcome no one knows yet.

Dinshah: That instrument that you have, then according to your opinion, has it any therapeutic or healing value or is it a useless piece of mechanism?

Hanor: Absolutely valuable. I should hate to practice without it.

When Dinshah had finished his direct examination, he turned Hanor over to Hagerty, but the prosecutor could not get Hanor to trip up in any way.

The next witness for the defense came to the stand. All in the courtroom trained their eyes on her as Dr. Kate Baldwin took her seat. Dinshah asked her about her medical training, her credentials and how she had become acquainted with himself and Spectro-Chrome. He asked her about the Spectro-Chrome equipment she had used in her medical practice. He presented pictures of Grace Shirlow, the girl whose clothes had caught fire and been badly burned, and asked her about the case.

"It was an absolutely fatal case," Baldwin responded. "In fact, I got that about 24 hours after the burn and the surgeon or doctor who had been called in, went out very legitimately, just simply wrapped it up in gauze and cotton to protect it, as he was quite justified in saying 'There is no use in trying to do anything with this!' In fact, the dressing was so tightly pressed into the raw surface that it was two weeks before I succeeded in getting it all off, as I would not force it off. I had to wait until the healing process took place, underneath and it loosened up, because if you pulled off the dressings you would pull off new tissues as well as old."

Dinshah continued his direct examination. "You did use this machine or a similar machine in connection with the treatment of the case?" he asked.

"I used it entirely," Baldwin said. "I said to myself, 'There is nothing in regular medicine or surgery that can make that child live.' Spectro-Chrome Metry was the thing I was working with at the time and I said to my assistant, 'We will see what Spectro-Chrome Metry will do.' That child had absolutely nothing but color and diet and dressing of sterilized waxed paper all through." She then went on to describe how the only setback there happened was when there was a case of diphtheria in the ward and health authorities, without her knowledge, had interns give injections of anti-toxins to every child in the ward including Grace Shirlow. The girl ran up a temperature of 105 or 106 degrees and was worse off in every way. Baldwin then tonated the girl with turquoise, blue, indigo and violet colors as Dinshah had taught her and that brought Grace's temperature down to normal.

Dinshah then asked Baldwin about other cases in which she had used Spectro-Chrome.

"What has been your experience in the use of the System?" he queried.

"Absolutely satisfactory. They will always need an undertaker. We do not claim that, you know."

"Beg your pardon?"

"We will always need the undertaker. We do not claim that we will not, but anything that is in human possibility, to be in normal shape, it can be done with Spectro-Chrome better than it can with anything else and with many, many cases, it is the only thing that would put the patient in a condition to function."

"Then, in fact, you will correct me, if I am wrong, that you are still using Spectro-Chrome stronger than ever?"

"I use practically nothing else."

"But Spectro-Chrome?"

"But Spectro-Chrome."

"Is the work, according to your viewpoint in a medical college, conducted along scientific grounds or merely as just a fake system to get money?"

"Absolutely most scientific thing there is in the healing art today," Baldwin answered.

It was now the prosecutor's turn to cross-examine Dr. Baldwin. Leo Hagerty rose from his seat and approached her.

He started out by grilling Baldwin about the Grace Shirlow case. He asked her about the waxed paper or paraffin used, about the special diet the girl was put on, what could be the direct cause of death from a burn like the girl had, and if she was a member of the American Medical Association.

"Have you abandoned the practice of medicine?" Hagerty asked.

"No," Baldwin replied, "I have not abandoned it. I use it if I have to but I shall not use it as long as I can get Spectro-Chrome. If I was cut out somewhere where I could not get Spectro-Chrome I would have to go back to the next best thing."

"You apparently have been convinced through the teachings of the Colonel and other things that Spectro-Chrome surpasses medicine?"

"I have."

"So that in your mind you practically have abandoned the practice of medicine?"

"Only if in a matter of emergency that I would use the old methods of treatment."

"How long have you been in that frame of mind?"

"Well, I commenced to use Spectro-Chrome the latter part of 1920 or first of 1921 and it did not take me very long to decide that it was better than anything else I had."

Hagerty seemed frustrated in his attempt to break the witness.

"And then, if I understand your testimony correctly," he continued, "you are of the opinion too, that Spectro-Chrome will cure anything and everything?"

"No, there was not anything on the face of the earth that will cure anything and everything. We have all of us got to die some time."

"Well, of course, I do not mean that. There is always a time when we are going to die. I am going to die. You are going to die, I suppose. What I mean, doctor, is that it will cure any of the so-called diseases?"

"Any of the so-called diseases, anything that is reasonably curable, it will cure and it will cure many things which drugs and general surgery and surgical work will not and surgical work will do better — cases of surgery will do better, if you use Spectro-Chrome in connection with it, than if you use only the old surgical method."

Hagerty then asked Baldwin if Spectro-Chrome would cure venereal diseases and tuberculosis. She replied that in her experience, it had.

"And will it cure cancer?" the prosecutor continued.

"In many cases of cancer, it will, if there has not been too much destruction of tissue, Spectro-Chrome will cure it, will build up the tissue. If it has to come to operation and there is a great deal of destruction of tissue, it will simply make them comfortable, for the rest of their lives, but, it will make them comfortable so that they can enjoy the rest of their life to a certain extent, without doping them with opiates."

"There are a great many world-recognized physicians who are attempting to find a cure for cancer, are there not?"

"Yes, it is one of the hard things that the medical world is trying to do and they have not gotten very far with it."

"But Spectro-Chrome will cure it?"

"I say Spectro-Chrome with - not an advanced case — will cure it, on the surface like the epithelium. I have had a number of those that were cured."

"And the medical world has always been looking for a cure for tuberculosis, too, has it not?"

"Yes."

"But Spectro-Chrome will cure tuberculosis?"

"Do you wish a case cited as ..."

"No, I do not care about going into specific cases. I am just asking your opinion about Spectro-Chrome. That is what I am getting at."

In answer to other questions Baldwin said she had had cases such as a strangulated hernia take the place of surgery, that she had used Spectro-Chrome to cure appendicitis as well as any toxic or septic condition. She said she had not been affiliated with any hospital for three years, and had ten machines set up in different treatment rooms of her office at 1117 Spruce Street.

The prosecution's witnesses included Dr. Albert Sy, a professor of chemistry for 36 years who taught at the University of Buffalo and various medical schools. Dinshah's witnesses included three physicians: Dr. Kate Baldwin, Dr. Manor and Dr. Martha Peebles, who had also been the Medical Inspector for the Department of Health in New York City for 20 years.

The testimonies given by each side were clever but Dinshah easily mastered his opponents. Dr. Sy, a highly recognized scientist, testified that colored light had no therapeutic value but Dinshah's cross-examination made him a spectacle, where even his university students that were present in the audience repeatedly tittered.

When Dr. Sy stepped down from the witness stand he breathed a sigh of relief and Dinshah felt sorry for what possible damage the professor's reputation might have suffered. But he compared Dr. Sy's plight to the famous Cardinal Thomas Wolsey of England, who in trying to serve two masters lost his life.

The trial went on for four days and then it was up to the jury to decide. Surprisingly, the jury deliberated for just a short time — only 90 minutes — before rendering its verdict: Dinshah was not guilty.

Dinshah heard soon after that Buffalo University where Dr. Sy was employed had given him a "vacation", and that a similar fate had been accorded by his employer to Dr. Reinhart.

Dinshah put things in perspective. Even though he had emerged victorious in the trial, it could have been destructive for him. He did not lose sight of that and knew also that rocky roads could lay ahead. Still, he was also aware of his near-impossible accomplishment over the previous decade. He was a man who assimilated in the American society of the 1920s who looked and dressed a world apart, and was of a different race, religion and nationality, and yet he amassed thousands of followers to an unbelievable healing science.

Dinshah's dream of making Spectro-Chrome available to help suffering humanity could still come true.

13

THE STATE OF DELAWARE GOES
AFTER DINSHAH

With Dinshah having emerged victorious from the Buffalo trial, one might think he would be optimistic about the future of Spectro-Chrome. He had total faith that his healing system was superior to that of conventional medicine, but he was wary that his opponents would continue to stop him every which way they could.

He recalled how years earlier, as his reputation grew far and wide from word-of-mouth, lectures and media coverage, his opponents, the "medical trust", ramped up its activity against him. In 1924, the American Medical Association, later joined by the U.S. Food and Drug Administration and U.S. Post Office, began what became a series of furious attempts to stop him. Dinshah once recalled: "from the day I presented that work to the world, untold privations, miseries and inconceivably illogical, heartbreaking opposition followed me at every step."

By 1932 Dinshah had been sent to prison seven times. A perennial opponent of the medical establishment with his Spectro-Chrome, which threatened the livelihoods of physicians and the pharmaceutical industry, Dinshah attributed his numerous unwarranted trips to prison to "an unprecedented frame-up of factions and rank perjury, through the nefarious machinations of those under his sledge-hammer activities."

Outside of the Mann Act sentence, which Dinshah proclaimed was a frame-up, most of his imprisonments could be attributed to him allegedly making fraudulent claims about a product or practicing medicine without a license. Despite his ineradicable belief in Spectro-Chrome, one would think Dinshah would yield to good sense and find a less controversial means of earning a living, but he was a bulldog of a fighter, and yielding was not in his vocabulary.

Determined as ever to carry on with his healing science, Dinshah continued giving Spectro-Chrome classes and lecturing. In his schedule were two free public lectures on his science at the Du Pont-Biltmore Hotel in Wilmington, Delaware. The first was to be held on Monday, October 10, 1932, and the second two days later, on Wednesday, October 12, both at eight o'clock in the evening. He mailed flyers advertising his lectures with the boldfaced heading: "Good News for the Sick! Vital Message to the Suffering!! Plug Your Health from the Light Socket!!" The ads promised they would be "illustrated with stereopticon, experiments and demonstrations." The lectures were offered "With the view of fully enlightening the suffering public on the matchless merits of this most efficacious and radical healing system, which in twelve years has been in use from the Atlantic to the Pacific Coast with unequivocal success in the normalation of all human disorders, including even the so-called 'incurable ones.'" The circular listed Dinshah's many honorary degrees including M.D., Ph.D., D.C., and LL.D., and it also advertised a free ten-day course "open both to professionals and laypersons with reserved tickets."

At the first lecture were hecklers who tried to disrupt Dinshah, but he was used to such behavior at his presentations and he continued his presentation undaunted. But some of his close associates let him know that a few physicians were in attendance and they felt that there was cause for concern about this. Unfazed, Dinshah just shrugged his shoulders. After the second class Dinshah returned to his home in Malaga, less than two hours away by car from Wilmington, but the following day he arranged to teach the advertised free ten-day Spectro-Chrome course in Wilmington starting a few days later.

Just after 6:30 p.m. on Saturday evening, October 22, 1932, about a week after his course had commenced, Dinshah and his wife Irene Grace arrived at the Odd Fellows' Building in Wilmington where he held his class in Rooms 304-306. Soon, a student, Martha Slaughter, came with her daughter.

Mrs. Slaughter explained that her daughter had been sick for years and had an "incurable" disorder. "What can Spectro-Chrome do for her?" she asked.

Careful not to examine the daughter or make any claims about his science Dinshah simply responded "Spectro-Chrome did many wonderful things in the past and properly used there is no reason why she should not be helped." Then he recommended that Mrs. Slaughter go to his Spectro-Chrome Institute in Malaga to learn more about his science.

The Slaughters thanked Dinshah and walked away. Dinshah left his wife to go to the restroom, and just as he returned and was putting on his velvet skullcap two men approached him.

"Ghadiali, we have a warrant for you," one of the men said.

"For what?" Dinshah asked.

"For practicing medicine without a license."

"I practice nothing, gentlemen."

Then Dinshah asked to see the warrant and one of the men read it aloud.

Dinshah's class was by this time waiting for him in the lecture room, but the two detectives, William Robinson and James Elliot, took him to the police station nearby. Dinshah inquired of the Desk Sergeant if he could give his personal property to his wife. The Desk Sergeant answered affirmatively, adding that otherwise all he had would be absconded, even his eyeglasses.

"I need them to see properly," Dinshah said.

The Desk Sergeant glared at him and responded "You will have nothing to see where you're going."

Having heard about Dinshah's arrest, Mrs. Slaughter came into the police station and inquired as to what had happened. She was told and offered to pay the $500 bail. A police officer advised her against it, saying Dinshah was a convict, but she said that at his lectures Dinshah had spoken about his oppression by the medical trust.

Dinshah was then led away and placed in a cell. Having no light, only a glare from outside prevented the small space from being pitch dark. He could make out two bunk beds, a sink and a toilet, but no toilet paper. As he wrote about his incarceration (in the third person):

> He did not undress or sit. He kept pacing the floor like a lion temporarily caged. He had faith in his innocence, faith in the Grand Architect of the Universe, whose protection was all the wealth he had. He trusted him in that hour of adversity in a city where very few people knew of him or of his labors in the service of mankind.

Lost in thought as he traipsed in his cell, Dinshah suddenly heard an officer shout "Come on doctor, you are going out!" Bail for his release had been posted by Mrs. Slaughter.

An arraignment was set for the following Monday and the officer warned Dinshah not to continue his free course. Dinshah asked to see a copy of the warrant and a captain, who was very cordial, showed it to him. Dinshah read that the arrest was made on a warrant sworn by a physician named William H. Speer, who was the president of the Delaware State Medical Society;

Dinshah was charged with violating Section 16, Chapter 27 of the Revised Code of Delaware of 1915, which essentially meant that he was in violation of the statute for practicing medicine without a license in the state. Dinshah observed that in the past the medical profession had "ambushed" him by not directly showing their influence in his arrests but now they were straightforwardly involved.

As reported in the newspapers the next day, Speer had contacted the American Medical Association about the lecturer from Malaga, New Jersey, who had come to Wilmington, and requested AMA's file on him.

At the hearing the complaining witness Spear spoke in a disparaging way about Dinshah, saying he was a charlatan who claimed he could cure disease with lights and that he cured a woman with tuberculosis with his machine. Dinshah denied he was practicing medicine in the state and said he was only lecturing, and for free. He said "I do not heal anyone. I do not practice medicine and I have a charter here which permits me to conduct lectures in this state for which no admission is charged." He pleaded that he was merely giving free lectures and that it was his constitutional right to do so. Dinshah offered into evidence a signed certificate from the British Consul declaring he was a doctor. A witness for the prosecution objected and Dinshah called out "I will never remove that title from my name. I am a medical doctor and I cannot change my title. If I am a king, I am a king forever."

Acting as his own attorney, Dinshah cross-examined William H. Speer with a steady stream of questions, apparently discombobulating him. "What made you bring this lawsuit?" Dinshah demanded. When Spears hesitated the judge said "He brought the suit to protect the interests of the public." Dinshah protested that the Court was putting words in the accuser's mouth. (Five people present at the trial would later send a notarized declaration to the County of Newcastle where the trial took place that "The attitude of the judge was plainly hostile to the interests of the defendant.") Dinshah's witnesses again included Spectro-Chrome's stalwart physician-champion Dr. Kate Baldwin and when the judge asked her if she was aware that Dinshah had been arrested in other states for practicing medicine without a license Dinshah objected; the judge then committed Dinshah to the Court of General

Sessions with bail set at $500. Once again, Mrs. Slaughter came through, posting the bail. After he was free, Dinshah asked Police Superintendent George Black and the Chief of Police George Boyd if he could continue his free course. They both said that if he did they could not stop someone from requesting a warrant on the same charge. That was good news for Dinshah. He thanked them and promptly returned to the lecture room where he picked up in his presentation of Spectro-Chrome from where he had last left off.

A new trial was set for Monday, January 9, 1933, and that day proved to be a busy one at the Court of General Sessions as it was hearing appeals of people accused of being Communists. Several armed police officers guarded the courthouse. Dinshah's case came up at noon, when Deputy Attorney General P. Warren Green announced that Dinshah was there for violating Delaware's Medical Practice Act. Dinshah stood; appearing in his native Indian dress with tight trousers and a skull cap, he caught the attention of all in the court room. Dinshah did not have legal counsel and the judge, Chief Justice James Pennewill, said: "If the defendant is not represented by counsel, the duty of the Court is to see that the Indictment is correct. This Indictment is not worded properly—there is no fee mentioned in it. The case is dismissed."

Dinshah was elated, but not for long. Dr. Speer obviously wanted to set an example that anyone who was not a licensed medical doctor could not practice in Delaware. As Dinshah walked out of the courthouse he was served with a new arrest warrant. Once again he was taken to police headquarters, and once again Mrs. Martha M. Slaughter posted his $500 bail.

The next morning Dinshah was arraigned. To his detriment the judge was the same hostile man as before. Dinshah contemplated requesting a new judge but decided against it, considering the vagaries of human nature. The charge was the same again — violating the stated Medical Practice Act — but this time it was amended insofar as Dinshah having "suggested an appliance for the cure of a disease with the intent of directly or indirectly receiving compensation therefore." At the trial witnesses appeared for the prosecution and the defense. A witness for the prosecution, Dr. George Vaughn smirked and laughed at Dinshah, who fired back at him so hard that the Court warned him to tone down his voice. Dinshah felt Judge Lynn's behavior was civil this time. He was released on $500 bail which was once again posted by Mrs. Slaughter.

Soon after Dinshah presented to the Supreme Court of Delaware a brief requesting redress on 46 grounds. He argued this Writ of Error for over two hours before four justices on the bench, but the Delaware Supreme Court sentenced Dinshah to pay a fine of $250 or go to jail for two months. In response, Dinshah filed a petition for a new trial.

Dinshah's petition to the Supreme Court of the United States was denied, without even a hearing, and he was ordered to appear on June 22, 1934 at the Court of General Sessions in Wilmington, Delaware. Appearing before Judge William H. Harrington, Dinshah was ordered to pay a fine of $250 plus $121.74 in court costs for a total of $371.74 or go to jail for two months. Dinshah paid the fine. With the cost of his petition to the U.S. Supreme Court running $595, he tallied his loss in the case to about $1000. Dinshah felt he was unfairly penalized for giving free public lectures in the interest of helping the sick. But at least this time he did not go to jail.

14

THE NATURALIZATION CHALLENGE

On Thursday, October 13, 1932, Dinshah, just having returned late the night before from Wilmington, was having a casual breakfast with his wife Irene Grace and their children. Dinshah took great pride in his five sons, and cherished the time he spent with them: Cyrus, born on October 25, 1924; Rochan, born on June 29, 1926; Darius, born on October 30, 1927; Jal, born on December 15, 1929; and Sarosh, born on December 26, 1930. The family's peaceful morning was suddenly interrupted when a man entered their dining room. He introduced himself as Deputy U.S. Marshal Buck and then immediately served a subpoena on Dinshah. Dinshah was astounded. He had no idea what it was for and he asked Buck, who responded that he could not tell him as he was not privy to the content of the subpoena.

The subpoena requested Dinshah to appear in a New Jersey District Court within 60 days to answer a bill of complaint against him. The subpoena made no mention of the reason for this and Dinshah was greatly puzzled as to what his offense could possibly be. He wrote to the signatory clerk on the subpoena who responded a few days later that a copy of the Bill of Complaint would cost $2.30.

Dinshah paid the cost and received the Bill of Complaint but the irony of the transaction did not escape him. He wrote:

> It appeared strange to me, that a super-wealthy Government like that of the United States of America, should order a man to answer a charge and then ask him to pay for information about the charge! I expected that common decency and good sense in Law would indicate that a copy of the Bill of Complaint should go attached to the Summons.

The Bill of Complaint, brought by the United States District Court of the District of Jersey, stated that the decree Dinshah had obtained in 1917 that admitted him to U.S. citizenship was "illegally procured" and that the certificate given to him was also illegally procured because he "is not of the white race, nor is he of African nativity or descent" and "by reason of his not being a free white person or a person of African nativity or descent is, and was ineligible racially for naturalization under the provisions of Section 2169, United States Revised Statutes."

The complaint actually went back to October 13, 1926 when an affidavit was filed by Henry B. Hazard, the Chief Naturalization Officer of the Bureau of Naturalization in the Department of Labor's Bureau of Naturalization which stated that Dinshah was "ineligible racially for naturalization" for the same reasons, and "that good cause exists for the institution of a suit under Section 15 of the naturalization act of June 29, 1906 (34 Stat. 596) to cancel the naturalization of said Dinshah Pestanji Framji Ghadiali on the ground that it was procured illegally."

Dinshah whimsically responded to the charges by writing:

> So I was not a White man and not a Black man either. I looked and looked ruefully at my skin — that unfortunate covering which brought me into Court once more. I rubbed it to see what was underneath, but do what I could, no color wave that I could

recognize as other than White, shone forth. I had presumed all along that I was White, of White father, White mother, White family, White ancestry, White nationality, White race, White through and through in fact, I was always a Mr. White and here comes Henry B. Hazard and swears that I was not White, although he never saw me or shook hands me.

Dinshah filed an answer to the complaint in which he identified himself as follows:

A Parsee Zoroastrian, a member of the White Race and is of Indo-European descent of the Caucasian stock Aryan Race and as such, fully eligible for naturalization as a Citizen of the United States of America under Section 2169 of the United States Revised Statures. The Race to which the Respondent belongs is the one that ruled in ancient Persia (Iran) and is recognized through history as the root of the present White races.

Dinshah wrote that the Naturalization Examiner and Judge William Seufert "after consent was secured from the high authorities in Washington, D.C." admitted him and:

for Henry B. Hazard to swear such affidavit as he made on October 13, 1926 is very surprising and distressing to me. Why the said Government Officer waited nine years before swearing such an affidavit and why the Complainant waited an additional six years before instituting the present proceeding is incomprehensible to the Respondent, who as a citizen of the United States of America relying on the integrity, sovereign honor and good faith of the Complainant, built an interstate humanitarian business which would be ruinously injured by granting the prayer of the Complainant.

Dinshah stated that the mere idea that he being born in Bombay would make him ineligible was not justified "on the obvious ground that an Englishman born in Africa does not become a Negro." Although he was born in India, he wrote, "he is a Free White person and racially eligible for citizenship under the law."

After this exchange of correspondence the matter of Dinshah's citizenship seemed to have subsided until early 1933 when he received a letter from the Department of Justice's U.S. Attorney for the District of New Jersey. Oliver Randolph, the Assistant U.S. Attorney for New Jersey requested Dinshah to send him his response to the bill of complaint which he filed on October 26, 1932, and that he come to his office to discuss the bill of complaint and the answer he had filed.

On the morning of Saturday, January 21, 1933 Dinshah walked into his Trenton office. When he arrived at the appointment he became surprised "when in a Black and White case," he wrote: "I found the Assistant United States Attorney, Oliver Randolph, a full-blooded Ethiopian!"

The two men spoke, and Randolph patiently listened to Dinshah's side of the case.

"I don't know how I am going to prove you are *not* a white man," the prosecutor said.

The story of Dinshah's naturalization plight made its way to the hearts of many Americans. The newscaster Lowell Thomas seized the story and broadcast it on his Columbia Broadcasting Company nationwide show. People from all over wrote letters to Dinshah. Several newspapers, local and in various American cities, reported the case, apparently in support of Dinshah.

On January 24, 1933 the *Evening Public Ledger*, published in Philadelphia, ran two articles in the paper in different editions. The *New York Times* published an article about the case, followed by an editorial the very next day supporting Dinshah and the contention he put forth:

even if he were a Hindu, the argument from ethnology and

philology would carry force. If anybody was entitled to belong to an Indo-European club it ought to be a native of India ... The courts will probably dispose of the case by side-stepping the scientific complexities, as they usually do. In the present instance there is no lack of ground for a decision. To go in for canceling citizenship right after a decade and a half seems neither justice nor common sense.

Numerous other newspapers reported on the U.S. government's action against Dinshah including the *Camden Courier-Post, Camden Morning Post, New York American, Vineland Evening Times, Philadelphia Record,* and a newspaper published weekly in Italian, *La Notizia.*

A veteran of being legally challenged or harassed, Dinshah felt the naturalization case against him was different than challenges in the past. As he wrote:

The situation was rather novel for me. It was so different from my prior experiences, when on my arrest for any false and perjurious charge, cooked up against me by the corrupt practices of the Medical Octopus or Ku Klux Klan, I could not even request attention to read my defense. This time, strangers, whose existence even unknown to me were drawn as if by magic. A woman lawyer from Los Angeles sent me some legal information. Several magazine editors gave their suggestions. American Civil Liberties Union offered to fight the case for me through their attorney A. L. Wirin. Naturally, I thanked all for their courtesies, but, informed all that I intended to fight my own case myself.

The naturalization case against Dinshah proceeded but it seemed there was one delay after another. He submitted whatever the Justice Department requested — information, documents, certificates, records, and even hoped that his compliance with the government's demands would result in the case being dropped. Some dates were set for the trial; first May 9, 1933, but that was cancelled, then six days later, May 15, but the Assistant U.S. Attorney Oliver Randolph cancelled that too, saying he was moving to have the case adjourned, with Dinshah's consent.

Dinshah returned a Consent of Adjournment but included a letter in which he reproved the government. He expressed his dissatisfaction with the trial date being changed without any reason given to him, and that an adjournment was made without providing him with a new trial date. "Unless the United States can prove that I am a Hindu and not a Parsee-Zoroastrian which I am, there is no case," he wrote.

Randolph wrote back that he requested the adjournment for Dinshah's benefit since he "had submitted some claims purporting to show that you are exempt from the provisions of the act" and that he "would let the Department consider your claims before going to trial with the case." Dinshah responded that although he was "puzzled" that the adjournment was made for his "benefit", that "no person wants to fight in the law courts and have his name dragged into the mud. I am neither anxious nor have I spare time to fight in courts of law, especially the very country which I have adopted as my own."

Three weeks later Harlan Besson, the United States Attorney for the District of New Jersey wrote Dinshah that "... after careful consideration of the matter, the Government takes the position that the matter should be submitted to the Court for its determination." Several months later Dinshah received a letter notifying him that the trial was scheduled for Tuesday, May 8, 1934.

On the designated date a trial was held at the Federal Court Building in Camden, New Jersey. The trail was presided over by the Hon. John Boyd Avis, United States District Judge. The prosecutor was U.S. Attorney Oliver Randolph.

Randolph proceeded to make the government's case that Dinshah was "not of the white race nor is he of African nativity or descent". Randolph cited the Thind case, 261, U.S. 204 that came before the Supreme Court from the Circuit Court of Appeals and which decided that Bhagat Singh Thind, "a high caste Hindu of full Indian blood, born at Amritsar, Punjab, India, is not a White Person within the meaning of Section 2169."

Back and forth the prosecutor and Dinshah went. "I shall show you that the Government has no case on which to stand," Dinshah said. He recalled a Naturalization Officer becoming inflamed that a man he disparaged as a "Hindu" should oppose him, and that he had lifted his leg and rolled up his pants to show him his leg so he would see he what race he belongs to. Then, Dinshah, with apologies for his brazenness, lifted his pant leg and asked the judge to touch his smooth skin, and the judge complied with his request.

Dinshah went on to list all his accomplishments since coming to the U.S., and stated that based on his citizenship, he:

contracted marriage with a girl of German descent, an American-born girl. She presented me with six sons. She would have been in the Court, but she has a baby in hand, Your Honor. On the strength of this citizenship, she embraced the Zoroastrian faith and what must have been in our mind affirmed at that time before a Philadelphia Notary Public, where I claimed I was a white man and my daughter brought in this country was a white woman. My wife is a white woman. If I were a Hindu, she would never have married me. You would ruin my family life, my business. Everything would crumble to pieces if my citizenship be taken away.

Dinshah spoke about how proud he was of his citizenship when he obtained it that when in public he branded himself as "the only Parsee Zoroastrian Citizen of the United States of America — America Always." He then showed the Court photos of his family — one with his sons, another with family including his wife. And a third with his children who had immigrated to the U.S., and their mother.

The judge focused on the latter photograph. Dinshah explained:

That is my first wife, Your Honor, the one who deserted me because I would *become* a citizen. Now, America throws me out and my second wife will desert me, because I did *not* become a citizen. The Government puts me into a funny situation.

Dinshah enumerated his commissions, memberships and offices he held in professional associations and then the certificates and diplomas he had received as well as honors, which were many: notary public in New Jersey; charters for his business from New Jersey, Illinois, Delaware, New York, Rhode Island, New Hampshire, Connecticut, Pennsylvania, Indiana, Ohio, Maryland; a Fellow of the American Geographical Society and the National Geographical Society; member of the American Association of Progressive Medicine; former vice-president of the Allied Medical Associations of America; president of the American Association of Spectro-Chrome Therapists; Flying Boat Pilot; graduate of the Curtiss School of Aviation; member of the American Association of Orificial Surgeons; and honorary member of the Hillsdale Fire Department. In addition, he said, he had "a truckload of European and Indian honors" which he decided not to present as evidence. He mentioned he had a quarter-million dollar plant that operated day and night.

Dinshah stated that if the government took away his citizenship it was nothing more than "a piece of paper to them, but to me it is all my life's work." He told how he came to America and served the city of New York as a commander of its Air Service, by being in charge of a police boat that received the Commander-in-Chief John J. Pershing returning from the war, and being a flyer for the city's police department. "There are certain other things that I did for the government about which I dare not speak," he cautiously added.

Later, Dinshah alluded to a more cryptic reason for the Court action:

I do not understand the motive of the United States Government, Your Honor, in dragging this case 17 years later. There *is* something behind it, and if somebody had gone in this chair we could have found out what the motive of the Government is; but I am left in the dark, somebody tries to stab me in my back and I do not know why the Government started this.

Dinshah next pressed his case that he was not a Hindu, mentioning that in the aftermath of the Thind case the American government initiated some 80 cases against Hindus in an attempt to deport them from the U.S. He then explained how Parsees are recognized the world over as white persons and "eligible to all European rights", granting them the privilege to ride in European railway cars in India and not the Hindu cars.

A recess was held but Dinshah stayed in the court room as it was his practice not to take lunch. An attorney observing the trial came over to him and after some small talk whispered: "You are going along all right. Follow the same line."

Dinshah gave some more history, quoting from books, then Randolph commenced his cross-examination. He asked Dinshah's residence from May 25, 1925.

Dinshah responded Malaga, New Jersey.

But Randolph brought up that he was convicted in a United States District Court.

Dinshah objected to the question saying it was "irrelevant and immaterial" but the judge told Dinshah that now that he was a witness it was relevant, since his credibility as a witness would be affected if he had a conviction. Randolph came down hard on Dinshah and Dinshah stated he had been "convicted of alleged violation of the Mann Act on the 4th of December 1925" and was fined for violating the Medical Practice Act in Cleveland, Ohio, in 1931, and for "practicing medicine without a license" in Wilmington, Delaware in 1933.

Randolph then asked if he was convicted in Rochester, New York.

"No, sir," Dinshah answered. "That was the case in Buffalo, New

York, before the Supreme Court of the State of New York. I fought the case myself and licked the medical doctors there. I was acquitted by the jury. That was what you call the Rochester case."

The judge looked at Dinshah. "That was on the question of practicing medicine?"

Dinshah shook his head. "No, Your Honor. They charged me with 'grand larceny' for selling fake machines and I proved the authenticity of the apparatus."

Dinshah felt the District Attorney did a good job in trying to destroy his reputation and that he would lose his civil rights. But he was also saving some key points and he was encouraged by the seemingly unprejudiced disposition of the judge. "May I request Your Honor to look at the Certificate filed in the Bill of Complaint of Mr. Hazard, the Naturalization Officer? There is a relevancy in the dates."

They affirmed that the date was October 13, 1926. Dinshah then produced his two-volume book *Railroading a Citizen*, which he said he had "published against my conviction for white slavery. I printed 2,000 copies of this and sent them from the President of the United States, the Attorney General, and everybody down the line about my 'frame up.' Who framed me?"

Dinshah asked the judge to check the date of the books' publication and then he presented them to the U.S. government. He put the books into evidence and said:

> I gave my whole story and demanded justice. I demanded redress and they were published on the 27th of May 1926. So Mr. Hazard woke up to get me out of this country now, after those were thrown in the teeth of the Department of Justice. It is *persecution*, Your Honor.

The judge then asked Dinshah about his conviction under the Mann Act.

They charged me with magic, hypnotism, mesmerism, Hinduism. The Mann Act is the transportation of a girl across the state line for immoral purposes. I had a girl secretary, who swore that she was in a hypnotic trance for ten months in my plant and because I was a Hindu I had 'magic.' It was with relation to my secretary across the state line.

"One individual?" the judge asked.
"One individual."
"You were not convicted of the business of white slavery?"
"No, no, only one girl charged me and I put this in issue here."
Dinshah went into detail about the charges, his incarcerations and his pardon by President Coolidge and then said:

If I am not a loyal American citizen, what am I? That is all in the files of the Department of Justice and the Honorable Oliver Randolph knows about it. This case came out of this Application to restore my civil rights. After three years, Your Honor, of reputable business, I filed the necessary affidavits to restore my civil rights. Instead of restoring my civil rights, they meant to kill me completely by taking away every spark of reputation I hold. Here is the paper.

The judge asked Dinshah about his other cases:

Certain factions who do not like my inventions have pursued me and persecuted me. It is all printed here. These factions, wherever I go for my lectures, tell the police department I am a convict of Atlanta and without any warrant they lift me out of my bedroom and lock me up for investigation.

"Where is this, in Delaware?"

This happened in Cleveland, Ohio. Before that they arrested me in

Rochester, New York, and tracked me to Buffalo, New York. There, the case went to the original side of Supreme Court of the State of New York, before Justice Thomas Noonan. Before a jury, I was convicted — I mean charged — with grand larceny by selling 'fake machines' and the jury by unanimous vote honorably acquitted me. I won that case myself without a lawyer. It is called the Buffalo case. I have papers in that case here. I won that case. Soon after, when I went to Cleveland, Ohio, they charged me again. I lectured among the public for my System and they locked me up for practicing medicine without a license. What do you think, Your Honor, the police department did there? I was before Municipal Judge Bradley Hull — a very fine gentleman — who heard the case very politely. There was a stenographer there, taking notes as this lady is taking them. I was led to believe that was a court stenographer. When he fined me, the judge put in a notation: 'I have the highest regard for this man, but for a technical violation of the law I am fining him $25 for breach of the medical law because he spoke about medical work.' That was all. I took no money from anybody. I never take money from anyone. I give free services. When I told the police to sell me the transcript of record to go on appeal they refused. I petitioned the judge to give me the papers and he refused to interfere and the police department refused to sell the transcript of record to go on appeal. Thus I could not go on appeal with the transcript. I went to the Department of Justice and said 'For God's sake, give me my pardon. This is William D. Mitchell's — the retired Attorney General's — doing. I cannot tell the inside, but if somebody from the Department of Justice had come here, I might have gotten it from those people'.

"You mean in this case?" the judge asked. "When was this Bill filed?"

A year and a half ago, but the affidavit is seven years old, Your Honor. Now, Your Honor, I went a year and a half ago to

Wilmington, Delaware, to the du Pont Hotel, to lecture on the Spectro-Chrome — my system of healing — that patented machine is just like a 'Violet Ray' machine. I did not see anybody, did not treat anybody, did not give any service and under a warrant — I mean with a warrant — that I practiced medicine without a license, they locked me up in the city jail. I was in eleven prisons, Your Honor, by this medical prosecution. This court has to protect me now, by restoring my rights, quashing this thing. Then I can go to Washington and tell the Department of Justice to go to the president and get my final release. It is getting unbearable for a man …

"What happened in Delaware?"

The chief justice quashed the indictment as charged. The moment I stepped out of the court they locked me up again. I pleaded 'double jeopardy.' The judge overruled me and after the trial gave me a fine with costs. I have been in eleven prisons. It seems to me like a motion picture performance, repeated. They fined me $250 and costs or an alternative of two months in prison. I carried out the appeal to the Delaware Supreme Court on 46 grounds. The strange thing is that the judges who sit in the General Sessions Court sit on the bench in the Supreme Court there. You are hit coming and going by the same judges! They threw me out there. Four days later I went to Washington, D.C. and then filed a petition for Writ of Certiorari in the United States Supreme Court to review the case. That case is pending. (That petition was later denied and a penalty was paid by Dinshah.)

After several more questions, Randolph wanted to call another witness, Henry L. Mulle, the Senior Naturalization Examiner at the Department of Labor.

Randolph asked Mulle if he had any "official records to show whether any proceedings were instituted to cancel the Naturalization Certificate of Mr. Ghadiali in the Southern District of New York."

Mulle said he had an original letter addressed to the Chief Naturalization Examiner, New York, dated October 25, 1923, and signed by William Hayward, the United States District Attorney, that referred to the cancellation of Certificate of Naturalization proceedings against a woman and two men, one of whom was Dinshah P. Ghadiali. He read from Hayward's letter: "I desire to inform you that on October 3, 1923 the United States Marshal for this District attempted to serve the above named respondents with a copy of subpoena but was informed that they live at the addresses given." Mulle said that in response to that letter a letter dated October 29, 1923 stated that the only address his office had for Mr. Ghadiali was 171 Madison Avenue, which came from the 1922 New York City telephone directory.

"Does your record show what was the final disposition of that case?" Randolph asked.

> A suggestion contained in a letter from Emory R. Buckner, United States Attorney, dated April 21, 1926, addressed to the head Naturalization Bureau, New York, stating that no service had ever been effected upon Mr. Dinshah P. Ghadiali and therefore he suggested that the proceeding instituted there be closed, because he could not locate him.

"What is the date of that?" Randolph said.

"That was April 21, 1926. I don't have anything here showing the discontinuance of the action."

Dinshah then took up the cross-examination of the government witness. He asked him when the Department of Labor questioned his naturalization after he was admitted in 1917. Mulle said 1923.

"Yes," Mulle said, "and very soon after the decision in the Thind case. The Thind case was responsible for the filing of a good many suits to cancel. They were instituted almost immediately after that."

"I see," Dinshah responded. "So your presumption, your official presumption is that the Thind case should be applied to everybody like me?"

"That is true."

The cross-examination continued for a while longer, and finally the testimony ended. Closing arguments followed, with Randolph starting. After a lengthy speech he concluded that "a high-caste Hindu, of full Indian blood, is not a White Person within the meaning" of the law, and "that the same conclusion from the reasoning" in the Thind case "would have been arrived at had Thind been a Parsee Zoroastrian instead of a Hindu."

Dinshah was impressed by the performance of the Assistant District Attorney, considering, at least, that the case was peculiar, hinging on the definitions of "free white person", "Hindu" and "Asian", and that all these elements were subject to the interpretation of Justice Alexander George Sutherland. He made a lengthy closing argument and finished up by saying his case rested on the doctrines of *Res Adjudicata* and *Laches*, and also the doctrine of *Equitable Estoppel*, which he had explained earlier. "You cannot deprive a man of what he creates on the strength of a contract on which he builds up a great equity," he said, "as I built it there."

The judge gave Randolph an opportunity to address Dinshah's argument of *Res Adjudicata*, which he did, and then he sat down. The previous din of voices uttering legal jargon and ethnology and history suddenly gave way to stone silence and an air of tension seemed to pervade the courtroom. Dinshah sat quietly, his vacant mien and stolid posture masking that he knew what was at stake here: everything he worked so hard to accomplish, his family, his dreams of changing the face of medical practice, would be harshly uprooted should the court decide in favor of the U.S. government.

At the bench, the judge, John Boyd Avis, held his clasped hands behind his neck and stared ahead, seemingly lost in thought. A former New Jersey state senator, he was 56 years old and nominated to be a United States District Court federal judge in September 1929 by President Herbert Hoover. No doubt, the legal mind of Judge Avis was consumed with pensive consideration of the testimonies and applicable laws and cases here.

Finally he broke the silence. "I think I can dispose of this case, without reserving decision on it, because, I think I have the facts and the law in mind, as fully now as I can get them. The real issue primarily, I suppose, laying aside all technicalities," he said, "is as to whether or not the Respondent was and is a White Person, as contemplated in the statute." He then spoke at length on his thoughts of this issue, concluding "I am inclined to think ... that the Respondent is a White Person, in the contemplation of the statute" and "that the Court has not the power at the present to grant the Prayer of the Bill of Complaint and cancel the Naturalization Certificate now held by the Respondent and as a result, I feel it is my duty to dismiss the Bill of Complaint. An order will be entered."

His eyes closed, Dinshah prayed silently to himself, and Randolph asked the judge to grant the government an Exception, which he allowed. Elated, Dinshah stood and thanked the judge for his kindness. "I am trying to decide in accordance with the law," the judge responded. "I am not deciding cases to do kindnesses."

The trial was over and the sound of chatter filled the courtroom. Newspaper reporters asked Randolph if he would pose for a photograph with Dinshah but he declined.

It had been a tough struggle, but as Dinshah himself adamantly asserted, his citizenship as an American was irrevocable and he was "officially a free white person". Newspapers jubilantly reported his court victory and the American Civil Liberties Union sent him a letter offering "Congratulations a thousand fold upon your success in beating the U.S. Government in its fight to cancel your citizenship and make you a 'man without a country'. You deserve additional congratulations because you handled the case yourself without the aid of an attorney and were successful in accomplishing what many attorneys have failed to accomplish." Many people were proud of what Dinshah had achieved for those whose liberty in the U.S. was at risk.

At the same time, Dinshah knew many of his adversaries had been keenly watching the proceedings, and while they must have been disappointed at the outcome, they would surely find other ways to stop him in his attempt to change the practice of medicine in America.

15

THE SPECTRO-CHROME INSTITUTE

Plato had his Academy, the French had their salons, and Dinshah incontrovertibly desired a similar illustrious institution for enlightenment and discovery, and for the dissemination of his beloved science of Spectro-Chrome. But unlike the shady meeting spots in the ancient Greek public gardens or the makeshift chambers in baronial mansions in the purlieu of the Jardin des Tuileries in Paris, the Parsee Indian-American needed ample grounds that could practically satisfy his needs of a scientific, cultural and humanitarian lab and retreat. In 1924 the burgeoning self-anointed medical pioneer's dream came true when he purchased a 23.23-acre parcel of land in the town of Malaga in southern New Jersey, and adapted it for his Spectro-Chrome Institute.

The grounds were like an expansive meadow on which buildings resembling 19th-century farmhouses overlooked the verdant terrain. Depending on where you were, stretches of flowers, grass or trees were in your immediate vicinity. Like a sprawling country manor, the Malaga Institute represented a significant upgrade from Dinshah's one-room office in New York City only a handful of years earlier.

Indeed, with Spectro-Chrome growing in the early 1920s —

despite the AMA's efforts to discredit it — Dinshah found that the needs of his central office outgrew its space. He set up a laboratory in Hillsdale, New Jersey and just a year later, in 1921, he established a base in Philadelphia in a three-story rented building at 1602 Summer Street. A year later again, when it became apparent that even more space was needed, Dinshah relocated his headquarters to 2401 North Broad Street in the city. But after traveling the country and attracting more and more new followers to his healing system, plus needing additional space for his experiments and development of new or improved equipment, it became apparent once again that another move to larger quarters, one that could fulfill the vision he had for Spectro-Chrome, was in order. That space was the Malaga estate.

Approaching across the flatlands, visitors could see the Institute from afar. Upon arrival at the locked steel gate they would call on a red-painted telephone in a box at the left of the fence that patched them in to the Central Office. Soon, the front gate would open and someone would come to greet them — sometimes Dinshah himself, to their pleasant surprise.

The Institute was open from 8 a.m. to 4 p.m., Monday through Friday. Visitors were advised to make appointments and smoking was absolutely forbidden on the premises.

The primary edifice of the Institute was the two-and-a-half-story Central Office and Research Laboratory. Its front door was flanked by several large windows on either side, and it had a white picket-fence porch before it. In front of that was a gravel walkway and an American flag, which, for many years, when Dinshah's civil rights were, in his belief, violated, did not fly.

The Central Office and Research Laboratory housed numerous rooms and areas: there was an office of the secretaries of the Institute and of the American Association of Spectro-Chrome Therapists; a reference library with stacks of books and a working table; a Lecture Room which contained not only equipment and chairs but an organ which Dinshah played; an auditorium which could hold up to several hundred people (its walls were adorned with Dinshah's numerous diplomas); and a dining room which strictly served foods in accordance with Dinshah's Rational Food of Man.

There was a spacious Office of the President with a 14-foot long desk on which rested stacks of papers and which contained shelves of medical, scientific and legal publications; offices for secretarial help were on the second floor. Nearby was a switchboard for long-distance calls. Till later hours of the evening someone would answer calls, and callers were often surprised to hear Dinshah himself welcome them. Several research rooms were also in the building: a Physics Room filled with an array of scientific apparatus for experiments; a Caloric Room to test attuned color slides; a Spectroscopy and Design Room; an Experiment Room filled with ultra-violet lamps, and infra-red light lamps machines and chiropractic apparatus which Dinshah tested for healing purposes; a Sanctum Sanctorum, Dinshah's sparsely furnished bedroom consisting only of a plain bed, dresser and chair; and a school room in the annex for Dinshah and Irene Grace's children to have their lessons.

Behind the Central Office and Research Laboratory were a Recreation Building, Engine House, and a Light Tower. On the grounds were also a carpenter shop, a printing plant, guest quarters, a garage to house the Institute's vehicles used for the transport of equipment and for Dinshah himself to drive around the country to teach and lecture, a gas-pumping station, and a park. In 1936, thanks to the approval of Gill Robb Wilson, the New Jersey Director of Aviation, a private airport beacon was installed at the Institute. As described in an issue of *Spectro-Chrome*:

> The beacon flashes in three distinct directions a beam of about four seconds of white light and about two seconds each of alternating red, green and violet light of the genuine Spectro-Chrome Attuned Color Waves, one complete round taking about thirty seconds. To comply with aircraft regulation, the beam is turned under the

horizon, yet makes an attractive and brilliant appearance for a long distance.

Some Spectro-Chrome Therapists predicted extraordinary things to come out of the Institute in this sparsely-populated location. Albert Greenham of Detroit, Michigan stated that "Malaga one day will be to Light and Color what Greenwich is to Time" and predicted that Dinshah's "new invention" would one day "surpass that of the great Ford Industry, which even only a few short years ago, would have been classed as wild dreams of its admirers and co-workers."

Visitors to the Institute were frequent, and if they were fortunate enough to come when the Spectro-Chrome originator and his family were there, they would be warmly greeted by Dinshah, his wife Irene Grace, and their sons. Visitors would say that at the Institute there was among the employees a resounding spirit of loyalty to Dinshah and such was their faith in his science that an ambience of doing something for the benefit of mankind pervaded the grounds.

In the carpenter shop young employees labored to build the cabinets for the Spectro-Chrome machines. Industrious and desirous of wanting everyone to obtain the benefits of Specto-Chrome, their mantra was "Shoot your orders and we'll shoot the works." The garage was not only a storage facility for the Institute's vehicles but a station for repairs, which were frequent given Dinshah's extensive traveling by motor vehicle. He was known to drive as much as almost 900 miles without stopping to eat or sleep or relieve himself. Beyond the gas pumps were transformers that provided electrical light for the Institute.

The Institute's Printing Plant contained sophisticated equipment for a small operation: a linotype composing machine, an intertype composing machine, a Miller high-speed cylinder printing press, an automatic Chandler & Price platen printing press, a Whitlock printing press, a Cottrell Pony cylinder printing press, a Dexter folding machine, a Liberty Folder, a Stereotype machine, a Chandler & Price power cutting machine, a Morrison stitching machine, a

Boston stitching machine, saw trimmer machines and a matrix-making machine.

In the Institute's garage was the so-called Spectro-Chrome Homecar, a virtual Spectro-Chrome Institute on wheels that Dinshah navigated to his various destinations. The truck housed a small office, equipment storage space, sleeping berths, a kitchen, shower, and lavatory. Its chassis was specially built and Dinshah would sometimes sit on a makeshift box when driving the vehicle (it was on the box seat that he drove the vehicle with the bare chassis from Detroit; when it was finished it had a full-width bench seat in front that was so wide that a passenger could actually sit on the driver's left).

For *Spectro-Chrome* magazine's January (Red) 1935 issue, Albert Greenham of Detroit, Michigan wrote of his visit to the Spectro-Chrome Institute and the time he spent with Dinshah:

> Here I had the chance to observe the man who had devoted his life to suffering humanity, asking nothing in return but just the opportunity to serve more freely; here is a man who has enough business capabilities to land him a first-class job in the business world without being harassed to death by a clique who thrive on human ignorance. Here is a man who has enough scientific ability to net him all the money he could use and keep him rolling in luxury if he so desired, if he wanted to use his ever-active, finely-constructed brain purely for self-aggrandizement. There is no knowing to what heights he would climb in the business or the scientific world and yet he chooses to sacrifice all these opportunities to serve you and me.
>
> Here is a man who endured the trials and tribulations of prison life in order that suffering humanity may be truthfully served. He has been laughed at, scoffed at, yea and I suppose even spat at, but still, in spite of it all he just continues to serve. How many men can you name in this world who would stand all this abuse for suffering

humanity? I personally could not name one, only the name of Colonel Dinshah.

Greenham likened Dinshah to both Jesus, who was incessantly harassed and humiliated but who was relentless in setting free the poor from exploitation even if it meant sacrificing his life; and David, who no match for the giant Goliath nevertheless embarked in battle, like Dinshah going up against "the Goliath of the Medical Profession".

As reported in the June (Turquoise) 1937 issue of *Spectro-Chrome*, none of Dinshah and Irene Grace's children attended school; Irene Grace home-schooled them all in the annex of the Central Office and Research Laboratory. The children all followed their father's tenets for good health so they were strict vegetarians and never had eggs, fish or meat, nor coffee, tea or tobacco. On June 13, 1937, at 9:45 p.m. Irene Grace and Dinshah's seventh son, Noshervan ("immortal soul") was born at 9:45 PM EST, weighing in at eight pounds.

On December 9, 1937, thirteen years after he purchased the grounds for his Institute, Dinshah paid off his mortgage. This came without any gifts or contributions.

Many had tried to silence Dinshah but in his fervor to make his science available to all, at this point, he refused to be muzzled. Indeed, despite his sundry arrests, imprisonments and trials, Dinshah wanted to reach out to even more people with what he felt was illuminating wisdom. In 1937, with donations from a fund he had started, Dinshah began construction of a non-commercial radio station at his Institute "strictly for educational and public service purposes".

16

DINSHAH RUNS FOR GOVERNOR

In the summer of 1937 Dinshah announced his candidacy for the governor of New Jersey. One of his campaign pledges was to end political graft. When the eldest son of the venerable Hindu non-violent political activist Mohandas Ghandi converted to the Mohammedan religion, Dinshah, an outspoken critic of alcohol and its damaging effects, wrote that the son, Harilal, now with the name Abdullah, "threw overboard his ancestral faith" because he was "drunk most of the time and in debt". Dinshah said alcohol was a "curse" to India and blamed the Roosevelt administration for repealing prohibition which he called a "boon" because the administration tried "to please graft politicians".

Dinshah ran on the independent-no graft ticket. To be on the ballot 800 signatures were required but as it turned out Dinshah obtained many more. His campaign theme was "Dinshah's Promiseless Platform" and it was printed on circulars as follows:

Because political promises made before election are invariably violated and the electors bamboozled thereby, I respectfully decline to make any rash and rosy promises at this time to secure the votes.

The State of New Jersey has been slowly and steadily gliding into a fearful political and economic mess because of graft and corruption on the part of the bosses and their henchmen.

As the Governor of this State, it shall be my duty to fulfill the will of the electors in every direction faithfully, fearlessly, and without regard to friendship or favor.

I shall zealously uphold that all will be in the interests of the people, my real employers. I shall give the public the best that is in me so the good of the public may be loyally served. I shall put forward my best endeavors to remove the causes of corruption and graft. I shall not play capital against labor or labor against capital, but shall show to both the way to genuine progress in harmony.

I shall in every possible direction so curtail the expenditures of the State Government that the terrible burden under which the people have suffered may be lifted.

Above all I shall place such machinery in motion as will remove the overlapping of ridiculous and unenforceable laws and simplify the legal processes so that the name of Jersey justice, once so famous, may stand before the world as an example of integrity of the highest order.

Since 1891, when I entered the service of the public, it has been my inviolate rule never to accept any gift, present, contribution, donation, tip, gratuity, inducement or token of any kind in the discharge of public duty.

I fear no one — only God above and conscience below and from them I have nothing to fear. This to the people of New Jersey I unreservedly pledge my word of honor that I shall serve them without regard to personal views, in a dutiful manner such as no party-elected Governor may expect to serve.

I do not promise anything — I shall fulfill what I say.

Nine candidates, including Dinshah, ran in the 1937 New Jersey gubernatorial election. The others were Lester Clee, Republican; A. Harry Moore, Democrat; John Kurzowski, Independent; Eugene Smith, Prohibition Party; John Butterworth, Socialist Labor Party of America; Frank Chandler, Communist; Henry Jager, Socialist; and James Murray, Independent Labor.

Dinshah was a serious candidate but pragmatic about his chances of winning. With his usual playful sense of humor, he even poked fun of his candidacy in *Spectro-Chrome* magazine with a piece entitled "Dining Room Fun" that had this dialogue between his wife Irene and their children:

Irene: Boys, your father is a candidate for Governor of New Jersey.
Cyrus: It will be good for the State.
Roshan: Yes, but he has no chance of winning against those Party Politicians.
Darius: Who is Lester Clee?
Hom: He is a Republican — Elephant!
Jal: And who is Harry Moore?
Hom: He is Democrat — Donkey!
Sarosh: And what is father?
Hom: He is Independent Vegetarian!
And Noshervan remained silent!

Longshots occasionally win political races and it couldn't have slipped Dinshah's mind how, if elected governor, his reforms would be received. With pledges of eliminating graft and corruption and bowing to the will of the people, it is easy to imagine him envisioning New Jersey becoming a model state under his leadership. He would institute reforms that would restore economic growth in the state, and all state employees would be impervious to the illicit pecuniary inducements offered by those seeking favors. That with the rampant political malfeasance in America, a Parsee from India who in his trustworthy, moral, incorruptible way guided the state to unprecedented success, would not only make New Jersey a paradigm for ethical politics, but show Americans — and the world! — that a one-time stranger in a strange new land — a non-native who worked hard and became an honorable citizen — could change things around for the better.

New Jersey's gubernatorial election was held on November 2, 1937, and the winner was the Democrat candidate A. Harry Moore with 746,033 votes, or 50.84% of the vote. Dinshah came in second to last with 1,264 votes, or .09% of the votes.

17

DINSHAH GOES TO INDIA

In 1939, thirty years after he picked up from his native country with empty pockets but a surplus of ambition to do benign service to mankind, Dinshah returned to India. In the three decades of his absence from his homeland, so much had happened in the course of his life that even he felt like it was an improbable real-life saga. The ambitious innovator had introduced a healing science to the western world that he had spent decades perfecting and which had attracted legions of professional health practitioners who had treated thousands of sick people who swore of its benefits; more than 5,400 of his machines were in daily use around America at this time; he had incurred the wrath of the American Medical Association and could only fathom what underhanded steps the organization as well as the drug industry who he also railed against may have taken to stop him; he had been taken to court several times for practicing medicine without a license and making allegedly false claims about his equipment; he had gone to prison for violation of the Mann Act, but exposed corruption in the prison and been granted clemency by a U.S. President; he had been jailed numerous times while awaiting arraignment; and the U.S. government had tried to rescind his citizenship several years after he had been naturalized as an American citizen.

Taking stock of his experiences Dinshah wrote of himself as he began his journey:

> He gains some, loses more. He determines to win, fighting the odds stacked against him, but no! at every move the loss becomes greater than the apparent gain. Time after time he finds himself penniless, starving, with numerous costly inventions yet uncompleted. He fights on — that Jupiterian soul never looks back. Slowly his projects take a nucleus; slowly does he find the path of usefulness opening before him. He toils on and on, working days and nights without stop and without rest. Years roll by and just as he expands his activities to the Service of Mankind, giving the best in him without grudge, a yawning chasm engulfs him and he disappears from the horizon of service for 17½ months. He climbs out, pursues the same path to which he consecrated his life. Again and again do his formidable opponents launch him into valleys of destruction, but each time he emerges unscathed, more determined to conquer. He continues to build, to spend, at all risks he goes forward.

For the upcoming trip, Dinshah had his Spectro-Chrome Institute pack 29 pieces of luggage of all sizes and painted blue to carry his Spectro-Chrome Metry equipment, since he planned to make demonstrations in India. With so much baggage conveying them anywhere presented logistical challenges but he made the 120-mile trip in the frigid weather from his home in Malaga to New York City in four hours.

It was Dinshah's habit to always look ahead and anticipate what obstacles might be encountered and he knew that it was important to account to customs what was going out lest he be challenged about what he brought back on return. So he brought with him a list of every piece of equipment being taken out of the country for his demonstrations along with a notarized affidavit that stated that no apparatus would be sold or given away. The contents of all his luggage were examined and accepted, and Dinshah then took his luggage along with the papers he was given and presented them all to the Chief Customs Inspector at the dock from where he was to leave.

His luggage checked in at the shipping line, Dinshah repaired to the Cornish Arms Hotel at 23rd Street and Eighth Avenue, a close distance to the steamship piers. The next afternoon Dinshah went to the Anchor Line's Pier 45 at the foot of West 24th Street where he boarded the 16,000-ton, 515-foot long TSS *Caledonia*.

At 5 p.m. on January 18, 1939 the *Caledonia* sailed out of the New York harbor heading for the Atlantic which it would cross to make its first stop in Belfast, Ireland. Dinshah was assigned to cabin 45, where in fact he would spend most of his time on the voyage since he adhered to a strict tenet of "no social relations with anybody." He even eschewed eating in the dining room so he could follow his rigid food principles and also work without being disturbed by other passengers.

Dinshah's daily regimen consisted of awaking before 5 a.m. and then beginning his day's activities: he would bathe, exercise, pray, then write until the time breakfast was served at 8 a.m. Then he would go to the Promenade Deck where he would walk a mile or so. By 10 a.m. he would return to his room, now cleaned and made up, and write for another couple of hours. Next, he would listen to the news on the radio, then, in the mid-afternoon, continue reading and writing. A few hours later he would take another walk, then have dinner around 7 p.m., and follow that by going to the movie that was shown each night on the trans-Atlantic voyage. He would go to bed at 10 p.m., except that he would read for three hours before actually turning in for the night. But he would not continuously sleep and when he awoke he would read, before turning out the lights again, only to awake for the day around 5 a.m.

On January 24, 1939 while on the *Caledonia*, news came on the radio that President Franklin Roosevelt had presented a health care report providing massive aid for federal and state programs "to improve national health".

Dinshah greeted the news with disgust; the President had noble intentions but could have made a better choice. Having anticipated a compulsory health care system that he deemed would serve to advance the interests of a privileged fraternity as well as being a tax drainer, Dinshah had presented to the American Congress "an unconditional offer to gift his entire American interest in Spectro-Chrome Metry and Spectro-Chrome Institute so the nation may be helped permanently without taxation that will prove a useless burden." Letters were sent out to every member of Congress and special requests for brief meetings in which the nature of the offer could be explained were sent to Vice President John Nance Garner and Speaker of the House William Brockman Bankhead. There was no response to Dinshah's heartfelt offer.

During the voyage Dinshah was treated as something like a luminary by the ship's crew. His reputation having preceded him, they were curious about him and engaged him in spirited conversations. The captain, Alexander Collie, was fascinated by His Highness the Maharaja of Patiala, and in Dinshah he found an informed conversationalist since in 1894 Dinshah had worked under him. The officers of the crew attended to their esteemed passenger's needs and provided all amenities they could to make his voyage pleasant. When the passengers on the ship found out who this curious man was, Dinshah was not shy in promoting Spectro-Chrome to them.

Nine days after the *Caledonia* left New York it arrived in Belfast, Ireland, and shortly after proceded to Glasgow, Scotland. Dinshah then boarded a train, with his luggage on board, bound for Liverpool, from which the next day he left for India aboard the *Cilicia*, another ship of the Anchor Line fleet that was launched on October 21, 1937.

Soon after leaving Liverpool, the sea became turbulent and caused seasickness in many of the passengers, who found relief (and warmth) in the ship's stock of liquor. Dinshah was never bothered by a ship's bumpy movements in shaky waters and he settled in by reading *Mein Kampf* by Adolf Hitler, whose evils he had already started writing about, and then other books. All the while the *Cilicia* moved on to other destinations: Gibraltar; Marseille; Port Said, Egypt. Aboard the ship the passengers frolicked with alcohol and cigarettes but Dinshah was holed up in his room and carried out many tasks, including indexing all the volumes of his Spectro-Chrome series so that readers may readily find information on ailments including case reports. At Aden Arabia, Dinshah found he was famous among its wealthy Parsee Zoroatrian community and through the courtesy of the family of Sir Hormusji Cowasji, he was personally escorted to the area's many points of interest.

Early on the morning of February 17, 1939 the *Cilicia* arrived in Bombay. Dinshah was received at the ship by his younger brother, Manekji, a photographer, and his daughter Manijeh and her husband Firoze. They were soon joined by a surprise guest — to Dinshah, that was — Jerbanoo Frami Jussavala, a woman who in 1897 Dinshah had successfully treated with color therapy, and whose case he had presented in 1920. As he would later write in his *Spectro-Chrome* magazine of seeing her, she was "an auspicious token of success for my healing system."

The greeting Dinshah received in Bombay was noteworthy. The editor of the *Digambar Jain* arranged for media coverage of Dinshah so Bombay newspapers of both the English and Gujarati languages ran stories of the heralded expatriate. Dinshah had become something of a local hero.

So austere was Dinshah in his abstaining from social relations that even though a wide gulf of time had separated him from seeing Manekji, he declined his brother's invitation to eat and lodge with him. Dinshah instead proceeded to the Bombay Central depot, and the next day he boarded the Bombay Baroda and Central India Railway which took him 162 miles north to Surat.

This is what Dinshah wrote on the response he received in arriving in the city on that Saturday afternoon:

The ovation and reception in Surat exceeded even Bombay. Heavy garlands and bouquets were piled on me by editors of newspapers, some former associates, some friends of former years, all enthusiastic at seeing me alive and energetic as a young man would be. After going through 28 years of hardships, horrors and imprisonments in America, they had portrayed the arrival of a foreign old fellow, bowed down with age, with a face drawn through misery looking as if he had been beaten down and was willing to croak; instead, out walked a quick-stepping, lithe and agile person, dressed in the old-time Parsee Zoroastrian costume, speaking with them and greeting each in the pure Gujarati language as if he had always lived among them! Their astonishment overtopped mine in many respects.

Mindful of his heavy workload ahead, Dinshah shopped for a residence for his three-month stay in the city and found one within the short span of three hours. It was a two-story house with 16 rooms that Dinshah rented for 195 rupees, or $65 for his sojourn in Surat. The next day he purchased all the furniture he needed for his stay and by the following day he had set up an office. He hired a domestic male worker to keep his house for 12 hours a day every day of the week at the rate of 21 rupees, or $7 a month.

Dinshah's started his day at 4 a.m. so he could turn on the knob for hot water. Two hours later he bathed, prayed an hour later, and then had breakfast at 8 a.m. The mail arrived early and even though he was new in town, the amount of correspondence was considerable. With word having gotten around that this celebrated American promulgator of good health was in town, bags of mail came beseeching Dinshah to treat babies and children and family members of all sorts. Dinshah regretted not bringing a secretary to help him with the volume of mail. The local pool of assistants was certainly affordable but hiring one would require training in the ways and methods of Spectro-Chrome for which Dinshah did not have the time.

As Dinshah later wrote:

> The rush of the sick was so exasperating that I had to advertise openly that I conducted no clinics but was in India solely for tuition in my science of Spectro-Chrome Metry. That began a howl of dissatisfaction and I was everywhere mobbed and pestered.

To fulfill the purpose of his trip, Dinshah summoned newspaper editors of the city and gave a four-hour demonstration of Spectro-Chrome that resulted in enthusiastic reviews, which of course in turn resulted in a bevy of inquiries about this mysterious healing science. With such an outpouring of requests, Dinshah rented the city's largest auditorium, the Annie Besant Hall, for a half-dozen lectures for eight rupees or $2.26 per night from the Theosophical Society.

Advertising the lectures proved not to be in the best interest of Dinshah, as the newspapers, thinking he was a rich American — weren't all Americans rich? — gouged their rates. Perhaps Dinshah made the mistake of inadvertently informing the Surat papers of the exorbitant American advertising rates so they felt that even though they weren't charging those rates their ambitious American visitor should be grateful that the rates they charged were considerably lower than what he would pay back home.

On February 26, 1939 Dinshah returned to Bombay to give a lecture on the principles of Spectro-Chrome Metry. In the audience was Sorah Palonji Kapadia, the editor-in-chief of Bombay's largest daily Gujarati daily newspaper, the *Bombay Samachar*. Kapadia's family was also present, including his nephew, Gave Kapadia, an editor of the *Times of India*. Then a freelance newspaper reporter, Jehangir Screwvala, arranged for Dinshah to speak at the Master School for Girls, where the audience consisted of a number of physicians. At the conclusion of the demonstration, Dr. Dara

Rustomji Hakim expressed interest in learning more about color therapy, and within a week ordered a Spectro-Chrome machine for his Racfad Clinic in Bombay.

Soon Dinshah went back to Surat where he printed advertisements for a Spectro-Chrome demonstration, which he gave on March 9, 1939. He was annoyed at the error of one newspaper whose ad in Gujarati about "attuned color waves" was supposed to read "Surman gothvela rangna moja" but instead was printed as "Suratman gothvelan rangnan mojan", which in Gujarati means "colored stockings arranged in Surat". It turned out that the embarrassing error had had no adverse effect as the lecture sold out and hundreds of people had to be turned away.

On the fifth evening of his demonstrations the editor of a weekly publication called Stri Shakti, or "Female Power", tugged at Dinshah and quietly said to him that his talk contravened the morality of Surat. Dinshah was taken aback. "Keep your ideas of morality in your pocket," he responded, "I know my business."

Once on stage, Dinshah opened up about puritanical views and the hypocrisy of the city newspapers which ran advertisements on venereal diseases and told of the ad touting a cure for impotence by a special pill bequeathed by a Mohatma on the Himalaya Mountains. Agitated by what he perceived as audacity by the Stri Shakti editor, Dinshah was in a state and railed from the stage, until some stood up to protest. Dinshah ordered them to sit down or leave, and the very man who incited him with the morality comment returned to his seat but an elderly man left in a huff. Meanwhile, the audience was getting worked up and as Dinshah lectured through the evening some members of the audience called out or made cracks while others shushed them. The disorder escalated to people breaking chairs, harassing women and chucking door handles out onto the street. At the conclusion of the demonstration someone turned out the lights so that there was chaos and disorder as the audience members tried to make their way out.

Ever-cautious about flare-ups at his public lectures, the next day, when Dinshah was being interviewed at a police station for a pistol permit, he requested police protection at his next lecture — the last of his Gujarati series. Perhaps because of word of the boisterous commotion in Dinshah's previous demonstration, a crowd flocked to Dinshah's next lecture, filling the hall quickly. Five officers were dispatched to the venue to act as sentinels. The volunteers who admitted the attendees were instructed to bar minor male youths from admittance but prior to mounting the stage Dinshah himself went row to row and plucked some 200 youths out of their seats and ejected them. During the evening one rabble-rouser stood and shouted out for Dinshah to apologize for the previous evening's disturbance, which resulted in others calling out, but when the police made themselves visible order was completely restored and Dinshah expressed his appreciation by announcing that he would extend the series for one additional evening. The next night several health professionals joined Dinshah on stage and at the conclusion of the lecture, the editor of the *Digamnbar Jain* placed a wreath of flowers around Dinshah and spoke words of gratitude to sustained audience cheers. A local branch of the Theosophical Society invited Dinshah to present Gujarati-language lectures on "Occultism and Higher Life", which Dinshah promised to deliver over five sessions along with his Manipadma theatrical piece, "Jewel In the Lotus".

Not everyone who attended the disrupted lectures, however, was willing to dismiss the brouhaha that had let out. Some complained to the District Superintendent of Police that Dinshah's discussion of the energy of certain colors was "indecent" and that Dinshah leered at one of the accuser's wives when moving his hands in certain ways.

Soon, a member of the Theosophical Society notified Dinshah that in order to comply with the integrity of the group he would have to refrain from using certain references. Dinshah was affronted, feeling that having been a member of the Theosophical Society since 1891 he had greater insight into the dynamics of the organization than all the members combined. He never delivered a speech with conditions attached or was dictated to and therefore cancelled the engagement.

Dinshah's blunt response struck a chord at the society and a member immediately came to visit him. Dinshah was told to please come and speak as his conscience desired and he willingly complied. A challenge, however, awaited him. Dinshah's stereopticon slides and his performance piece were in English but he was told that his audience would mainly consist of Indian women who did not understand the language. So in only four days' time he had to revise all the slides in Gujarati, which he worked around the clock to do.

The first lecture was presented at six in the evening on Sunday, March 26, 1939. Many seats in the hall had been extracted and the women sat on the covered floor. All the seats were removed for Dinshah's next lecture and a capacity crowd of 2,000 sat on the floor. For his last event hundreds of upper-class families were unable to get tickets to Dinshah's dramatic performance piece, so great was the demand. After the series, Dinshah was deluged with invitations for more presentations but respectfully declined owing to planned activities for the rest of his visit.

Dinshah wanted to speak at the Framji Cowasji Institute in Bombay where he had launched his career as a scientific lecturer in 1891 when he was just 17, and which therefore occupied a tender spot in his heart. A journalist acquaintance of Dinshah requested arrangements and Dinshah subsequently received a letter requesting 25 rupees for rent for each engagement plus five rupees for lights with a required deposit of 50 rupees and the balance to be paid at the engagement. Requesting seven dates in early April, Dinshah sent in over 100 rupees.

There was no immediate response to Dinshah's reservation but finally a letter came from the honorary managing trustee of the organization, saying that Dinshah was short on the rental and should have remitted 350 rupees for security. Dinshah wrote back saying he had merely followed the directions of the original correspondent and added that he had worked with the trustee's father many years ago and that he hoped that his brand of health practice wouldn't be a problem for him. He wrote that because he sensed otherwise. The trustee, Dr. Framroze N. A. Moos, was a graduate of a London medical school and the director of the Gokuldas Tejpal Hospital in southern Bombay.

Very shortly after Dinshah received his money back with a letter stating the Institute would not rent to him. His demonstrations, the letter stated, were not of "public interest".

Despite the cancellation of this planned lecture series Dinshah was not at a loss for filling his time. He was invited to preside over the birthday celebration of the great Jain Master, Mahavira, at the Annie Besant Hall, named after the British activist who supported Indian autonomy. The celebration was a religious event and Dinshah thought the Jain Committee's regard of his traditional theosophical views, anti-slaughter promotion, and support of a vegetarian lifestyle made him a proper choice to lead the ceremony. An overflowing crowd filled the hall as the event commenced at 6.30 p.m. on April 2, 1939. The audience of men and women sat on the floor and invited delegates spoke in the Hindi and Gujarati languages.

Dinshah himself spoke in Hindi and Gujarati and to the delight of the audience interspersed Shlokas verses of classical Sanskrit poetry. He spoke against slaughter and invoked examples of other religions, the Lord Mahavira Swami and Gautama Buddha. Before the ceremony concluded, the group unanimously passed a resolution requesting the government of Bombay to honor the Lord Mahavira Swami by making the calendar date Chaitra Sudi 13 a public holiday for the 1.2 million Jains in the Bombay Presidency. As the leader of the event Dinshah submitted the petition to Balasaheb Gangadhar Kher, the Prime Minister of the Bombay Province.

Now into April, Dinshah was anxious to enlighten the citizens of Bombay, his beloved birthplace, about the science he had devoted years of his life to promulgating in America. Dinshah's first presentation was on April 9, 1939, his first public appearance in his city of birth in 36 years. Early in the evening he mounted the stage, which had American flags at the sides. He saluted the American flag projected on the screen behind him and began his lecture in Gujarati. As always, Dinshah spoke not from any prepared script but extemporaneously. He liked to follow what he deemed was the Socratic method of lecturing — that is, to walk the podium from side to side and make eye contact with members of the audience in a way that made each person feel like he or she was the focus of the speaker's attention. By looking at the audience members and feeling their aura he could determine what he should or should not say or what alternative direction he should go in. Dinshah's demonstration lasted two hours and the audience, charmed and fascinated by his presentation, applauded frequently.

All his lectures in the series went smoothly except for one instance in which a woman occupied the seat designated for the *Times of India* in the area reserved for journalists. Dinshah informed her that the seat was reserved and said he would provide another seat in the hall for her but she became indignant and left.

In his last presentation Dinshah announced that in upcoming lectures in the city the following month under the authority of the government of Bombay he would speak on why his healing art prohibited the use of alcohol. Several students he had encountered in Surat, knowing he was a teetotaler, had requested him to address the subject of temperance. Dinshah was ever-cognizant of the sensitivities of the millions of people in India, but little did he imagine, however, the impact of his announcement! Just the mention of alcohol was like lighting a powder keg.

In India, Dinshah traveled to different hospitals to look into their practices. At one hospital he examined its rates which were printed in the Gujarati language, which was not a problem for him at all since it was his native tongue. The rates were in rupees; at the time one rupee equaled 35 American cents. Some of the items Dinshah translated were as follows: appendicitis operation: 50 to 100 rupees; hysterectomy operation: 50 to 100 rupees; tonsil operation: 20 rupees; hernia operation: 40 to 50 rupees; ovarian cyst operation: 50

to 100 rupees; kidney stone operation: 50 to 100 rupees; consultation fee at the hospital during hospital hours: 2 rupees; blood examination: 2 to 5 rupees; tooth extraction without injection: ¼ rupee. While these rates would be affordable to Americans, Dinshah was bothered by them since in India the wages were extremely low. As an example, he brought up that in the country a male domestic laborer worked for him for the going rate of 20 rupees a month, which in U.S. dollars would amount to $1.63 a week. He hoped that with his drug-free Spectro-Chrome science, the poor would get the medical help they needed.

No matter where he was, Dinshah maintained his wry sense of humor. For his *Spectro-Chrome* magazine he wrote for the May (Green) 1939 issue:

> Some fortune-teller of Calcutta, India claims to have made a "fluid", which if applied to the human body would render the person invisible. He refuses to demonstrate it until an antidote be invented to make it reversible, because, he states that his fluid applied acts only one way to permanency. That inventor does only have to offer that fluid for sale to me and I shall gladly present him with all I have, if his chemical will make the American Medical Association invisible, provided solely that the Reversibility Fluid should not be permitted its invention or application. The same active fluid may well be used for the Bombay Medical Council — in fact, for all the medical affiliations, it will prove a real blessing to the sick world.

In India, Dinshah set up a satellite Spectro-Chrome office in Surat. It was in the same location where he had had his Electro-Medical Hall and Apakshapata Printing Press up until the time he emigrated.

18

DINSHAH AND PROHIBITION IN INDIA

Following Dinshah's announcement of his lectures on prohibition the Parsee Zoroastrian newspapers in Bombay censured him. Normally, Dinshah did not back down from the subject matter of his lectures but the remonstrations were so great that he asked the students who had requested lectures on alcohol abstention if they wouldn't mind if he spoke on another topic. The students agreed and Dinshah delivered a lecture on "Life In America". The meeting was held in Gandevi, a town in the state of Gujarat whose ruling prince was the Maharaja Gaekwad of Baroda. The lecture was successful with Dinshah responding to questions about marriage, widows and social customs in America with levity that left the audience in stitches.

Dinshah's main purpose in traveling to India was to introduce Spectro-Chrome to the country. He had sold three Spectro-Chrome machines in Bombay and eight in Surat, with the promise of more purchases, when the anti-prohibition newspapers ran disparaging articles about him and those who had promised to purchase machines backed out. But Dinshah needed to provide instructions to those who did purchase the machines — among them five medical practitioners, a dental surgeon, a therapist and a law student — and that is what he did in what he called a "special meeting" that ran from Saturday, April 29, 1939 through Monday evening, May 1, 1939.

Prohibition was a contentious issue at the time in India and as much as Dinshah had resolved to stay away from it, he had become engulfed during his relatively brief sojourn there.

A decree had been passed providing for the removal of alcohol from liquor stores and bars in Bombay and its surrounding areas on August 1, 1939. There were plans for enforcement officers to take inventories of liquor shops and bars which they would seal off for excise agents to later remove the inventories to government depots. It was expected that there would be demonstrations and riots in the street once the law took effect.

Invitations poured in from dozens of clubs in India for Dinshah to speak. With a reputation for being brilliant in the areas of health and science, the subjects he was called to speak on varied. But with prohibition the hot topic in Bombay, it was hard for him to avoid the issue. In the audience of a speech he gave in Surat on "Occultism and Higher Life" were some members of the Theosophical Society who remembered Dinshah speaking on the harm alcohol could cause some four decades ago, and they beseeched him to lecture on temperance in anticipation of the new prohibition law going into effect.

Dinshah did not want to get involved since he was no longer an Indian citizen but expressed the view that if he was officially invited by the government of Bombay then he would accede to the invitation. Several hundred respected residents of Surat signed a petition requesting Dinshah to give an address on prohibition and it was delivered to the Minister for Public Health, Dr. Munchershah D. Gilder, a prominent physician who was once the president of the Indian Temperance Association and who seemed to inherit his penchant for abstinence from his father who had served as an officer in the Temperance Association and who in fact had enlightened Dinshah himself into temperance when he was 18 years old. While Dinshah was in Bombay giving demonstrations on Spectro-Chrome, an appointment was made for him to meet with Dr. Gilder and around the same time, through the efforts of a friend, another meeting was set up for Dinshah to meet with the Chief Minister of Bombay State, Balasaheb Gangadhar Kher.

At two o'clock in the afternoon of April 11, 1939, Dinshah paid a visit to Chief Mininster Kher, who received him amicably. Their discussion turned to prohibition and the Indian leader expressed his sentiments that Dinshah, now from America which with its 21st amendment had its own nationwide prohibition of alcohol, would be the perfect man to lecture on alcohol abstention in India. Dinshah again expressed the view that since he was not an Indian citizen any longer that it would be out of place for an alien to speak on the contentious subject of prohibition but if he received an official invitation from the Bombay government he would be happy to do so. The chief minister concurred and the lectures were set to run, one on each day, from the 9th to the 11th of May.

Although Dinshah was a Parsee Zoroastrian by birth it was the Parsee Zoroastrian newspapers in Bombay that lambasted him most (Parsees are not generally teetolares or vegetarians). The first paper to attack was the daily Gujarati-language *Jame-e-Jamshed*, which half a century earlier had praised Dinshah in editorials and articles like he was an illustrious and distinguished scientist, but now went after him every way it could, maligning his Spectro-Chrome, his background and his inventions. If the paper was aiming to hit a nerve it struck a bulls-eye by branding Dinshah a charlatan and a prevaricator, and maligning his credentials. It brought up Dinshah's incarceration for the charge of transporting an underage girl across state lines. As Dinshah would later write in his monthly magazine "*Jame Jamshed* belittled me until it made me into a man of straw, a braggart, a boaster, a downright boob of no learning or merit."

The next Parsee newspaper to mount the disparagement bandwagon was the weekly journal, *Kom Sevak*, which translates as "Community Servant". Published in Gujarati, the publication thoroughly besmirched Dinshah personally and his Spectro-Chrome.

Nasarwanji Navroji Engineer, the weekly's editor, had attended Dinshah's Spectro-Chrome lectures and Dinshah had subsequently monitored the paper so his denunciations came as no surprise. But so acrid was his invective with charges that Dinshah deemed were patently false that the Spectro-Chrome originator regarded the articles as libel and said he would have sued if it hadn't been for the fact that he had to shortly return to America.

While the Parsee newspaper smears were gnawing, Dinshah now had the pressing matter of delivering the temperance lectures he had arranged with Chief Minister Balasaheb Gangadhar Kher. On the morning of Sunday, May 7, 1939, Dinshah boarded a train at Surat and arrived in Bombay early in the evening. He left his luggage with the station master and immediately checked in to the Regent Hotel. With the Parsee newspapers inflaming their readers with calumny against Dinshah and his stringent prohibition platform, coupled with the liquor trade's obvious dismantling by a temperance law, it was easy for Dinshah to surmise the acrimonious greeting he would receive at his government-sanctioned anti-alcohol Bombay speeches. He notified political leaders as well as the Prohibition Propaganda Board of his concern of clashes and disturbances and was assured that order would be kept.

At 6 p.m. on Tuesday, May 9, 1939, Dinshah was picked up in a car with Assistant Secretary Bachoo Bhansali and driven to the Sir Cowasji Jehangir Public Hall in Bombay. By the time they arrived a huge crowd had gathered. Dinshah and Bhansali were met at the platform entrance by Kanaiyalal Maneklal Munshi, Bombay State's Home Minister and chair of the event who had a distinguished reputation as a barrister and Gujarat literary figure. Together they walked to the platform entrance under the piercing eyes of the crowd.

The air was thick with tension and Dinshah sensed the crowd would not just be rude but disorderly. A half-hour after he arrived Dinshah mounted the platform with Chairman Munshi, the Prime Minister's Parliamentary Secretary Gulzarilal Nanda, Prohibition Propaganda Board Assistant Secretary Bachoo Bhansah and reporter

Jehangir Screwvala, and the crowd began hooting and hissing and shouting out "Boycott Ghadiali!" and sundry other epithets. Then spectators started pelting the speakers with eggs, fruits and other objects and it seemed like all-pandemonium had broken out.

The speakers stepped away with the notion that they would give the crowd time to release its disgruntlement, which they felt was instigated by interests of the liquor trade, but when they approached the microphones again after ample time it turned out that the crowd was not any less bellicose. Pellets of one kind or another accosted those who moved forward to speak and the shouts of the crowd made their intention clear: they wanted Dinshah removed.

The police were ready to intervene if needed but as Munshi made clear to Dinshah, "non-violence" was the way of the city and law enforcement would only move in if the crowd perpetrated any kind of physical violence. Dinshah respected the idea of non-belligerence but also felt the crowd had an obligation to be civil at a public event. He did not make his personal feelings known as he was just a guest and remained tacit on the subject.

An hour went by, then another, and then another. Still, no respite from the rambunctious group. The assemblage was being photographed and filmed, all at once. There would be a permanent record for the media to show of the halted proceedings, and as Dinshah thought, of the unruliness of the mob. People shouted lewd comments about female kin of the speakers and some even exposed themselves brazenly. Dinshah was duly ashamed that the group was composed mainly of his own kin, Parsees, and he lamented that this revolting behavior was all borne out of the inextinguishable desire to imbibe liquor.

Chairman Munshi finally had enough of the unruliness and directed Dinshah to proceed with his presentation. "Your honor, I don't think my voice can carry over that of the shouters," he said. "If you quiet them a little I shall willingly speak."

Munshi cast off Dinshah's reticence, responding that if Dinshah were just to begin with his slides then that would be enough to calm the crowd. He assured Dinshah that they were prepared for any contingencies that might arise.

The lights dimmed and the first slide, of an American flag, projected onto the screen. As the image appeared a more raucous clamor was heard on the left side. Undeterred, Dinshah proceeded. Part of his presentation was on evolution and when pictures of frightful monkeys appeared Dinshah compared the ruffians in the audience to them. Pictures of other animals flashed on the screen and using gestures, Dinshah compared himself to them, like the lion, to which he signaled to his chest his own strength. This went on and on and as the crowd grew more incensed Dinshah thought he was fighting violence with "non-violent violence".

The topic of Dinshah's next lecture at the Sir Cowasji Jehangir Public Hall, given the following day, was "Alcohol: Its Effects on Man." Well before the lecture was to begin the streets outside the hall were overflowing with people, many of them Parsees. The hall filled up quickly and those who were late were denied admission. The latecomers plowed into the barriers but volunteers rushed to stave them off. The Parsees demanded their "rights" be respected and soon a rumble broke out with fists and chairs. The police arrived and arrested a number of people. Order was restored and Dinshah delivered his speech.

On the third and last day of Dinshah's trio of lectures at Sir Cowasji Jehangir Public Hall, all Parsees were barred entry due to the outbreak of fights on the two previous days. It was believed that many of them were connected to those who would gain by keeping alcohol legal. The speech went smoothly but what gave Dinshah the most satisfaction was seeing that those who were out to smear him were defeated. The print media including *Jame Jamshed* and *Kom Sevak* ran many false accusations about him and tried to bring him down but they couldn't. If the most powerful cartel in all the world could not, that being the American Medical Association, then certainly this bunch could not. Dinshah prided himself in striking back at them with powerful words. He criticized his foes for invoking the Grand Master Zoroaster in the context of possessing wine— not even a real wine but a juice — for the purpose of creating indestructibility, which he deemed an outright lie. Alcohol, Dinshah asserted, should not be consumed by people.

And with his final speech at the hall Dinshah concluded his trip to India. At 7:45 in the morning of May 12, 1939, several police officers from the *Cilicia* police department accompanied him at his request to the Ballard Pier for the return to America. While he thought he was well able to handle himself should he be attacked by anyone who opposed his views, Dinshah didn't want to be involved in any kind of altercation that would prevent him from returning home while his numerous bags made the trans-Atlantic voyage without him.

As it turned out, several newspaper reporters were on hand to question Dinshah on prohibition, which was to be enforced in Bombay starting on August 1, 1939, after he boarded the *Cilicia*. Dinshah said if he was wanted he was willing to give his services as an intrepid and incorruptible civil servant for free to the government of Bombay to make prohibition successful.

"Will prohibition succeed in Bombay?" a *Times of India* reporter asked. "Surely it will succeed," Dinshah wryly replied, "if they will succeed in keeping out bribery, corruption and graft."

The decks were crowded and the police thought it prudent for Dinshah to not remain visible so they requested he repair to his cabin, which he dutifully did. Early in the afternoon the *Cilicia* set sail and slowly Bombay faded in the distance. With Dinshah having been appointed an American correspondent to the largest Gujarati-language daily, the *Bombay Samachar*, he kept busy writing dispatches supporting his views and positions which he mailed when the *Cilicia* stopped first at Port Said, Egypt, and then at Marseilles, France.

On May 31, 1939, the *Cilicia* dropped anchor in Liverpool, England, and from there Dinshah proceeded by train to Glasgow. To avoid the long inspection process of British customs with his voluminous baggage containing all his scientific equipment, he commissioned an entire train car to carry his baggage which got a customs seal when it was placed on the car under official supervision. After the train arrived at its destination, a customs officer accompanied it to the *Cameronia*. On the evening of Friday, June 2, 1939, the ship left Glasgow and headed for the Atlantic Ocean. Heavy fog and icebergs slowed it down, but it arrived in New York City only one day late, on 12 June, 1939.

It was an exhilarating if not exhausting trip for the self-proclaimed medical healer, and as he headed home to Malaga, New Jersey after clearing customs, he knew there was much work to be done with Spectro-Chrome. He just didn't know what to expect from the various forces out to stop him.

19

DINSHAH RETURNS TO INDIA

Only five months after Dinshah returned to America he left for India again. He was not vindictive by nature, but he felt his reputation had been unfairly tarnished by those in the media in India who did not like his advocacy or abstaining from alcohol and that he deserved to have his name cleared. So he decided to circle the globe again to sue two newspapers — the daily *Jam-e-Jamshed* and the weekly *Kom Sevak*, as well as his former wife for the allegedly libelous articles she wrote about him, and a rich liquor entrepreneur, Sir Byramjee Jeejeebhoy, for defamation also.

Before Dinshah set out he penned a couple of brief articles in his *Spectro-Chrome* magazine about the benefits of his healing science for India. In the December (Scarlet) 1939 issue he wrote:

> Because of the war in Europe, the Government of Bombay, India, is also facing trouble dealing with profiteers." He pointed out how pharmaceutical companies, with drugs in shortage and the demand for them high, stockpiled drugs and jacked up their prices. He went on to list needed drugs from acetylsalicylic acid and its salts to X-ray chemicals and implored the Bombay government to

investigate Spectro-Chrome as it would find most of the drugs on the list unneeded and "by the use of which India can be independent of profiteering and the lives of the suffering public may be saved, without socialist or communistic regimentation. The less government in business, the better the business.

In an article in the magazine's November (Magenta) 1939 issue entitled "Need of Spectro-Chrome in India," Dinshah pointed out the high costs for drugs and injections in India and stated: "the real profiteer is the medical doctor." He concluded by saying that:

> looking at all this from the standpoint of Spectro-Chrome Metry, if our Science and its Equipment be introduced into Hindustan, all cries of profiteering would cease and the local industries which produce electric power would be materially benefited. I shall be glad to place my resources at the disposal of the Government, should they give me a hearing and accept Spectro-Chrome as the logical way out of ailments.

At 9 p.m. on Saturday evening, November 4, 1939, Dinshah set out from New York City on the SS *President Harrison* of the American President Lines. His wife and all his children as well as some fellow workers were on hand to see him off. After arriving in India, Dinshah promptly repaired to the Court of the Chief Presidency Magistrate to file libel suits against the editors of the two newspapers, as well as his ex-wife Manek, for alleged defamatory articles she had published under her name. The suits were heard before a justice, Indravadan N. Mehta. Subsequently, retractions were issued.

As reprinted in Spectro-Chrome's August (Indigo) 1940 issue, here is the *Jam-e-Jamshead* piece, entitled "Clarification of a Grave Injustice":

When Colonel Dinshah P. Ghadiali returned to India from the

United States of America in February 1939, we were the first to give publicity to his various scientific activities. However, later when he spoke on the subject of "Alcoholism", our views being different from his on the subject of "Prohibition", we published certain adverse articles in which he was referred to by us as "Jailbird", "Masquerading as Colonel", "Bogus Colonel", "Fraud", and so on.

Since his return last month from America to India we had the opportunity of examining a large number of documents and photograms pertaining to his ramified activities. All these documents we found to be duly verified by the Secretary of State for New Jersey and the Governor of New Jersey, authenticated with the Imperial Seal of His Britannic Majesty and the signature of the British Consulate General.

From these we are satisfied that the objectionable references that we made about Colonel Dinshah were unjustified and groundless. We found that in 1918, Colonel Dinshah was Surgeon Captain in the New York Police Reserve and Governor of the New York Police Aviation School, later being promoted to the rank of Colonel and Commander of the Pioneer Wing of the New York Police Reserve Air Service. For his loyal services the city of New York authorities presented him with the Victory Medal, after the close of the Great War.

Our personal remarks against Colonel Dinshah must have caused him great pain and we take this early opportunity of withdrawing the said imputations and expressing our sincere and heartfelt regrets for the serious injustice done to Colonel Dinshah.

Being personally approached with such retraction by the editor, a youth of about 28, out of sheer kindness looking to the future of Ardeshir and not desiring to have it blasted sentence by sentence, Dinshah requested the Court to mark the case as "sufficient gratification received out of Court" and had the accused acquitted. Later, Dinshah filed a suit in the Bombay High Court against the proprietors and editor of the *Jam-e-Jamshed* for civil damages to the extent of Rupees 100,000 and Rupees 20,000 costs. Summons being served on six defendants, the plaintiff deposited Rupees 1,200 with the High Court as security for his appearance.

Dinshah also sought to file suit for libel again his former wife, Manekbai Hormusji Jamshedi Mehta, who had had several articles published with her byline in the Parsee-Zoroastrian-owned *Kom Sevak*. She had deserted him in America, and she was difficult to find in India, but after a diligent search she was located at the Taj Majal Hotel in Bombay. It had been 27 years since he had last seen her. The wound of the desertion never healed, and seeing her malicious statements about him in the newspapers abraded his emotional scar even harder. Confronting her face-to-face was difficult, and seeing her all those years later, the glow of her womanly youth was gone, her softness of face and feminine beauty diminished. Now, the woman he once passionately loved in the tenderness of her youth and had last seen nearly three decades earlier, was an elderly, haggard version of her former self, and Dinshah could not help but feel pangs of pity for her. Nevertheless, he personally served a summons on his ex-wife and when she appeared in court she brought a handwritten apology which the Chief Presidency Magistrate ordered her to read aloud. Dated April 5, 1940, it was reproduced in *Spectro-Chrome*'s August (Indigo) 1940 issue as follows:

Virtuous-named Colonel Dinshah Pestanji Ghadiali, Bombay: You executed summons on me for that I humbly pray that before you proceed pay attention to this letter and save this afflicted one from further affliction.

I came from America to India of my own will leaving your protection; the twenty-seven years since then I passed in intense unhappiness. From the misunderstanding by which I came away and the separation from you and the children, my mental condition became unstable. I did not see anything in proper light. When you came to India in 1939, at that time others instigated me that you did not divorce me according to the Parsi Law hence a charge of "bigamy" could be tenable against you. Then I also got a letter from Nasharvanji Navroji Engineer, the Editor of *Kom Sevak*, that he would have convenience in printing should I write against you.

Through the result of my own error, I had come to India, yet I felt that I made you unhappy. By such thought I made the grave error of having printed in the *Kom Sevak* a series of articles making against you serious imputations. I did you intense injustice and greatly damaged your brilliant reputation and career. Those writings were finished in seven issues beginning 25th June 1939 ending on the day of 6th August 1939 and by then I believed some pressure would be applied on you. All the imputations therein I withdraw unconditionally and apologize.

The people who instigated me, those people did not have information that you had sent me legal summons from America and gotten my signature.

Also the second marriage you contracted after waiting for me over nine years and receiving competent Divorce. By the false inducement of folks and the instigation of the Editor of the *Kom Sevak* what evil I wrote about you and the pulverization I made of your reputation among the people for that I am intensely repentant. I know by my experience that you possess the noble virtue of generosity and forgiveness so depending on that virtue accepting my cordial apology do not have me sentenced in my present fallen aspect by proceeding with the case, because I am not able to bear such affliction. Receive my blessings by giving me pardon with the former pure love forgetting the past incident with generous heart.

May God Almighty be your protector.

Hearing his former wife's contrite words had a deep emotional effect on Dinshah. Subsequently, he asked the court for a settlement in her case. As reproduced in the August (Indigo) 1940 *Spectro-Chrome*, his petition was as follows:

May it please your Worship, Now comes the complainant before the Worshipful Court and prays:

That the hearing of the case was set for May 22, 1940.

That meanwhile, the accused tendered the complainant the unconditional apology in Gujarati, herewith attached with its translation.

That the soul-stirring terms in which the said unconditional apology was couched and the contrition shown by the accused for the past, touched the heart of the complainant, more so as the accused was formerly his wife.

That the complainant accepts the said unconditional apology as sufficient gratification for the offence committed.

That the accused is now present in the Court.

That therefore, the complainant requests the Worshipful Court to record the said composition and mark the case settled out of Court.

For such kind courtesy the complainant will ever pray.

Most respectfully submitted.

Dinshah Pestanji Ghadiali, Complainant.

Dated: Bombay, Tuesday, April 9, 1940.

Dinshah wept as both Manekbai's unconditional apology and his petition for composition were read aloud. His emotions overpowered him and he was unable to keep in check his usual equanimity and aplomb. The Court asked him how he would like the case resolved. "What else can I do, your Worship? She was once my wife." The magistrate considered Dinshah's plea, and acquitted Manekbai.

Dinshah soon left for America — there was something important he had to do there — and his criminal libel suit against Sir Byramjee Jeejeebhoy was dismissed, according to law, because of his departure although he was free to institute it again if he returned to India, and he did indeed have intentions of returning. Therefore, before he left he filed civil suits against two other individuals and set up an office at

Ahmed Manor, Warden Road in Bombay for the advancement of Spectro-Chrome.

Dinshah was anxious to return to America as he planned to file his nomination for the election of Governor of the state of New Jersey. He had run once before and lost, but thought he should try again. With his vast experience of serving and leading in governmental and quasi-military organizations in the U.S., and his penchant for honesty and incorruptibility, he felt he would make a fair leader of the state where he resided. However, the 66-year-old Dinshah arrived in the U.S. from India on June 16, 1940 and was informed by New Jersey's Secretary of State Thomas A. Mathis that the deadline for filing the nomination petition for independent candidates had been May 6, 1940. No nomination could be filed after that date.

With his lawsuits unresolved and determined to see Spectro-Chrome spread in India, Dinshah once again decided to return to the country of his birth, intending to travel on the *President Harrison*. However, a steadfast censurer and abstainer of drugs, Dinshah refused vaccinations and cholera inoculations so the American President Lines told him the *President Harrison* would only take him as far as Japan. He beseeched the Java-Pacific Line to take him to his destination and the company agreed to take him on a steamer, but only on the provision that he obtain a visa on his American passport from the Japanese and British consulates. Dinshah succeeded in doing this, and bought a ticket for the steamer. With these arrangements made, he purchased a train ticket to San Francisco from where he planned to depart.

But an obstacle came his way. Dinshah was informed that in order for him to make the trip he had to have his American passport validated. He sent it to Ruth Bielaski Shipley, the Chief of the Passport Division, and after a long stretch of time had passed he was told there was no valid reason for him to go to India, and that his passport had been "filed" away. He requested it back and it was refused; he then traveled to the Passport Division in Washington,

D.C. to take care of the matter personally. He was told Shipley was not available and that he would only be permitted to travel abroad if he had "urgent business" to attend to such as purchasing needed materials for the United States government. Dinshah demanded his passport be returned and it was — with punched holes and a stamp reading "Cancellation" on it.

20

METAPHYSICS AND DINSHAH

Restricted from traveling again to India, Dinshah now resumed his attention to his color-healing science and the activities of the Spectro-Chrome "planet" chapters spread around America. One aspect of his personal background that he didn't blare, but which he also didn't hide, was his metaphysical side. He in fact wrote about it genuinely and straightforwardly in his *Spectro-Chrome Metry Encyclopedia*, and even credited it with leading his way to Edwin Dwight Babbitt's *Principles of Light and Color*, the book which he said was his initial inspiration for investigating colored-light healing.

As he tells the story, Dinshah befriended the son of the landlord of his boyhood house at 92 Parsee Bazaar Street in Bombay. Sometimes the two chums would spend a couple of hours together in the evening delving into deep philosophical discussions. One evening, his friend, Dinshah Phirozshah Sethna, casually mentioned a *Times of India* article which told of members of a group called the Theosophical Society who reported having communication with "Masters" who were lodged on the Himalaya Mountains. Dinshah thought this was absolutely absurd. "Oh, there must be a telephonic connection," he laughed. "How can anyone talk a distance of 1,300 miles?"

Yet something about the story intrigued him and that night he couldn't sleep.

Unable to let go of this preternatural tale, the next day Dinshah decided to investigate for himself what was behind it. He visited the Theosophical Society's Blavatsky Lodge on Hornby Row, and encountered the secretary, a bearded Parsee Zoroastrian named Munchershah Shroff. Dinshah observed Shroff to have a sober mien, and wrote that he greeted him "with a peculiar Ahem-ahumph that sounded like the neigh of a horse." Dinshah proceeded to pose questions to the secretary, whose speech was interfused with those curious Ahem-ahumphs. The puzzling sounds notwithstanding, Dinshah was fascinated by what he heard. The Society secretary told him that it was indeed possible to communicate with people distances away without the aid of any device by means of "occult processes". Several distinguished persons had already investigated this communications phenomenon and found it to be veritable. There was Sir William Crookes, the British chemist who invented the Crookes tube; Helena Petrovna Blavastky, the Ukrainian-born occultist; William Thomas Stead, a British writer and editor who pioneered investigative journalism; and Sir Henry Steel Olcott, an American journalist who had investigated the Spiritual movement. Dinshah cogitated these inquiries. If these noteworthy people could be open to a rationale for the occurrence of strange phenomena, then it was worth looking into for himself.

Shroff gave Dinshah various materials to study, and Dinshah went home and carefully read all he was given, and then contemplated the notions behind it all. Having more questions, he returned to the Society and after obtaining further information was inducted as a Fellow of the Theosophical Society on October 26, 1891.

What attracted the 17-year-old Dinshah to the occult (which at the time referred only to hidden knowledge and not devil worship as it later came to mean) was that previously he actually had experienced odd incidents and strange things — hidden phenomena, perhaps — but never questioned the "causes" behind them. He had performed experiments of hypnotism on his mother and grandmother, which with the propitious results gave his family members the heebie-jeebies, and he considered that he might actually have a special propensity in this medium. "Many a time, inexplicable incidents occurred," Dinshah wrote, but the clincher for him happened when he was 14 years old.

As a young teen Dinshah did odd jobs to fund his love of experimental research, and one day he painted an inch-thick wooden signboard and affixed it to the window outside his father's room. When his father saw it hanging there the next day he became infuriated and crashed it to the floor. When it didn't break his temper exacerbated and he smashed it into his son's neck. Dinshah's fiber was such that his love and respect for his father was unconditional but when he saw blood pour out of his mouth he himself flew into a rage, seized his father by his arm and flung him onto his bed. "Scarcely did this happen," Dinshah recalled, "when a resounding slap from an invisible hand fell on my cheek and in a moment I realized the wickedness of my action. What penalties that one rash act brought into my life may never be known to the uninitiated."

This unsettling incident propelled Dinshah to investigate the cabalistic side of life further. He was now a member of the Theosophical Society, which had, as he observed, three fundamental objectives:

To establish the nucleus of a Universal Brotherhood without distinction of race, sex, caste, creed or color; to promote the study of comparative religion and philosophy; to investigate the psychic powers latent in man. The first object I always favored, having an utter dislike for snobbishness, ceremonials and pomp; with the second I was in accord, having already gone into it; the third appealed to me because it pleased my ticklishness for research and from investigation of the psychic powers latent in man it was easy to drift into the investigation of self. I soon found what was there and oh, what discoveries awaited my thirsty mind!

To Dinshah's delight, the Theosophical Society had a substantial inventory of books and pamphlets on the occult sciences and he satiated his appetite for information on this subject by reading as much as he could from the collection. One of the books he found was Edwin Dwight Babbitt's *The Principles of Light and Color*. He perused the tome with a sense of enthrallment. In this book he found there was a "beautiful message" and he wondered if the medical establishment could have missed something in its erudite inquest into the healing arts. Dinshah subsequently launched himself into serious contemplation of the mysteries of nature. Nature was magnificent, he apprehended, nature was grand, but locked away in it were secrets and enigmas that with the right imagination and scrutiny could be discerned.

Not long after, Dinshah had another experience which confirmed his belief in occult processes. It was late in the evening and he had been reading *Researches in Magnetism and Odic Force* by the celebrated German chemist Carl Ludwig von Reichenbach when he put the book on the table next to his bed, on which a coconut oil lamp rested, to go to sleep. He awoke at 2 a.m. and noticed both the oil lamp and book that had been on the table were no longer there. The oil lamp was in an elevated recess in a wall that his father had designated for it and the book was on the floor. Having been in a slumber he thought his mother had come into the room and for some reason moved the items away. He got out of bed and retrieved both the oil lamp and book and placed them back on the table. To make himself drowsy he picked up the book to read, and then fell asleep again. When he awoke an hour later he found both the oil lamp and book had moved back to the same spots. He considered that his mother or another family member had come in his room and moved the items. He fetched the oil lamp and book again and the situation repeated itself. Then something happened which bewildered him:

> I leaned over to get the volume, on which a small black animal was scratching. Barely had I touched the book when a dazzling, brilliant Aurora spread before me, my consciousness changed from the Physical Plane and I became clairaudient and clairvoyant. Two persons were evidently talking, though separated by a great distance and through the process of interception, my consciousness crossed their etheric path. I heard and saw. The final words, "A Mahatma is a Raja" sank as if seared into my Higher Centres and soon a sable pall pervaded the visual horizon. I awoke from the Trance.
>
> The next day I talked about this incident to an intimate friend of mine, Kershaspji Rustamji Modi, who was also a Fellow of the Theosophical Society. He told me that some day I should have the solution of this mysterious event. In the first week of December 1891, I went to Adyar, Madras, India as a delegate of the organization and there in the shrine when I went for prayers I not only saw the picture of one of the persons whose conversation I heard, but personally met the other party.

Any qualms Dinshah had about the occult were obliterated by this unaccountable experience and consequently he hurled himself into investigating human latent powers. He found the results to be astonishing, and he decided to take what he learned and apply it to curing the ill and infirm.

21

———————————————

MORE SPECTRO-CHROME PRAISE

By the early 1940s, no physician, osteopath, dentist or chiropractor could openly practice Spectro-Chrome Metry in the U.S. without fear of losing his or her license; not just Dinshah was pursued by legal authorities for treating people with Spectro-Chrome, but licensed medical doctors and others as well. Thus, with the threat of legal action heavily hanging over them, many licensed health professionals who practiced Spectro-Chrome healing therapy felt compelled to stop using it altogether even though they felt they successfully treated their patients with it.

But not all health professionals stopped using Spectro-Chrome; they were just now forced to use it in an "underground" way — to use it on the hush-hush, so to speak. And for those who continued to use it in this climate where any practice but that of conventional medicine could invite the attention if not legal action from law enforcement, they could no longer submit case histories and testimonials for publication in *Spectro-Chrome*. For case histories and testimonials the magazine became the province of laypersons and perhaps health professionals who used pseudonyms or not their full names. Outside of the Planet officers, whose full names were printed, most laypersons became identified by only their first names and the first letter of their last name, or their initials.

Despite laypersons even being at risk for practicing Spectro-Chrome Metry, there were many who simply refused to stop using it and they continued to be active members in their local Planet organizations and also in submitting results with Dinshah's colored-light therapy to *Spectro-Chrome* magazine. At a First Detroit Planet meeting held at the Hotel Tuller in Detroit Spectro-Chrome affiliates gave case reports. These were reproduced in the January (Red) 1940 issue and included the following:

Jessie N. reported (1) a woman with a very serious disorder had gone to Mayo clinic. Apparently there was no hope for her. She purchased a Spectro-Chrome and after using it two years, finds no trace of the disorder. (2) A woman suffering from phlebitis and confined to bed. Green turquoise and magenta were used. After one week she was able to walk.

Sara C. reported (1) a child with scarlet fever. Spiroscil (breaths per minute) 40, Kardoscil (heartbeats per minute) 140. Turquoise, blue and magenta were used. After three days, Spiroscil 32, Kardoscil 130. Child is recovering. (2) Child with impetigo, ears and chin covered with sores. Tonated with lemon systemic, turquoise systemic, magenta on Area 4 and child is normalated. (3) Mother of Sarah C. had cold, Kardoscil 100, Spiroscil 25, was dizzy and had sore throat. Turquoise systemic, purple on Areas 2 and 3 were used. Cough was gone in two tonations. Now using green and magenta. (4) Sara C. had a cold and run-down condition. Kardoscil 100, Spiroscil 12, pain in Areas 18 and 19. Turquoise systemic, orange on Area 17, now feels very well.

Adolph D.'s sister-in-law was deaf in one ear. The other ear started to pain. The ear was filled with wax. Green cleared that condition. Orange, red and magenta were then used and her hearing is now perfect. Effie D.'s son-in-law was hoarse and had a stiff neck. Two orange tonations and the cold was entirely gone. On other occasions, he was at home for week with same disorder.

In the same issue of *Spector-Chrome*, Lydia D. of Merrill, Wisconsin told of her nephew who was sick with a throat problem and not able to eat for six days. After the second tonation he started to eat. A sister had second- and third-degree burns, had turquoise atcowa [attuned color wave] applied once a day and the pus was cleared within a week. Then blue systemic was applied once a day for two weeks and new skin formed. "Sufferer is very grateful to Spectro-Chrome," Lydia D. reported.

Then there was the pharmacist from Milwaukee, Arthur D., who was introduced to Spectro-Chrome and subsequently ordered equipment and books and voluntarily wrote:

Spectro-Chrome Training Course is a wonderful insight into the medical folly which I personally thought was the 'profession.' I am thoroughly convinced of the complications and superstitions used to fool the public and am thoroughly disgusted with the power of the American Medical Association in this supposed free United States of America ... The Home Training Course ought to be studied by the medical doctors and they would realize their folly; but they are duped by the AMA and cannot release themselves from their bondage to that Association.

The next issue of *Spectro-Chrome* was likewise filled with case histories and other assorted pieces. Here are excerpts from a letter from Ruth B.D. from Mound City, South Dakota:

I am sending you testimony (unsolicited), telling you what Spectro-Chrome did for me. Please accept it as a token of my appreciation.

I am another one of those persons who tried Spectro-Chrome as a last resort. Consequently, recovery for me was retarded. However, slow improvement is much better than none at all.

I am a rural school teacher, 2 1 years of age. At the close of my second term of teaching, my ankles started to swell and I began noticing a feeling of persistent fatigue. The medical doctors told me I had nephritis. Three different doctors could do nothing for me except "diagnose" the case and declare it "hopeless and incurable". At the end of 2 ½ months of medical "care", my body was so swollen that I could no longer wear any clothing; my eyesight was so blurred that I could not tell the time when the clock stood six feet away from me; my appetite was gone; my blood was so weak that on the hottest days of July I had to have a hot water bottle on my feet in order to keep them warm. My Frontelim [urination] was discolored and the quantity reduced to practically nothing.

Finally, on the nineteenth of July, 1939, I began taking Spectro-Chrome tonations, renting the equipment from a friend. The first two green tonations showed a change in me. My eyes, which had previously watered continually, stopped watering. After taking three tonations each day for several days, the accumulated poisons, which I had taken in the form of medicines, began passing through the bowels. On the twelfth day, my bowels moved so often that I lost control of the number of times. This removal of poisons continued at various intervals for five months, the swelling disappearing at the same time. In three days, my Kardoscil was reduced from 90 to 80; the Spiroscil retained at 18. In a week's time my feet began warming up by themselves. The Frontelim increased and became normal. My sight and appetite also returned. Although I felt fine, I remained in bed most of the time for five months, because I still had some swelling.

During the eighth month I began appearing in public, to the astonishment of those seeing me. They heard that the medical doctors sent me home to die. I live in a small village, so my illness was "the talk of the town". One man said, "What can that light do for her?" Well, they soon found out and it was a glorious revelation to many, as well as a great boost to Spectro-Chrome.

A friend who had used Spectro-Chrome for years gave me tonations each month. After that, I improved enough so that I could read the Specto-Chrome Home Guide and with advice from her occasionally I "became my own doctor", using the greatest invention in history. Green, turquoise and lemon systemic were used with orange on Area 8 and magenta scarlet on Areas 4 and 18. After the swelling disappeared I used orange, yellow systemic, with scarlet local.

With thanks to Spectro-Chrome, I can again look forward to returning to State Teachers' College this Fall. Words cannot express my feeling of admiration and gratitude towards Spectro-Chrome.

Successful treatments of all types of diseases and ailments continued to be reported in *Spectro-Chrome*. Letters were printed in which users praised Spectro-Chrome equipment as "worth its weight in gold" or a "miracle machine". There were sections in which Dinshah answered questions from practitioners or commented on some area of interest or concern, for example, "Sunshine cannot produce the precise results of Spectro-Chrome"; men who complain that a nagging wife can cause a heart disorder should be aware that men can cause an adverse effect on women by finding fault with them; that sports like football and hard ball baseball should, after "very careful analysis and serious consideration", be avoided or modified so as not to cause injuries; "Spectro-Chrome Metry will in time wipe out other systems of healing, especially medicine and dentistry and destructive surgery. It is not the *coming* remedy, but *is already* come 21 years and is impossible to uproot or upset."

In the issues there were almost always reports of Planet meetings with case histories given by their affiliates; often the affiliates effused praise about the results they got with Spectro-Chrome but sometimes they spoke of frustrations of one sort or another. For example, at a meeting of the First St. Louis, Missouri Planet held at the Hotel Melbourne in St. Louis on April 4, 1940, the Deputy, Clemens M. P.

Neumann proudly announced that he was able to get a Spectro-Chrome machine in the Barnes Hospital to tonate a woman who had a bad streptococcic infection in her throat. He received permission from officials at the hospital to install a machine but he wasn't sure if it was a "step forward or backward".

Neumann tonated the sufferer with turquoise and she began to perspire. While he was waiting to tonate the sufferer with magenta a half dozen physicians came in the room and asked him what he was doing and he responded that he was waiting to irradiate the person's heart. The doctors, as reported in *Spectro-Chrome*, "looked at him like he was crazy and should have his head examined." They forbid him from administering any more treatments and Neumann left "discouraged", although the sufferer's husband said he would have him tonate his wife after she left the hospital and returned home.

In the October (Purple) 1940 issue of *Spectro-Chrome*, there appeared an interesting piece of information about the late Dr. Kate Baldwin, the former senior surgeon at Woman's Hospital in Philadelphia and, following her successful results with the healing science, one of its most strident champions. Baldwin had witnessed numerous calumnies against Dinshah and observed his reputation being severely tarnished by the American Medical Association in its *Journal* and, being curious about the occult which was a subject of deep interest to Dinshah, had engaged a female psychic in California for a numberscope of Dinshah. Dr. Baldwin revealed not a single detail of Dinshah outside of his birth date and this was the response she received, as printed in the Purple 1940 issue of *Spectro-Chrome*:

Birth Path: November 28, 1873
 Sign of the Zodiac: Sagittarius
 Birthstone: Turquoise
 Colors: Green and Chestnut
 This Birth-Path denotes a soul brave, imperious and rash. Although generally calm, things that annoy him, excite him greatly. Although not vindictive or spiteful, he will end a friendship for all

time, when right to do so. Born to give orders but not to obey them. Fond of discipline and method is everything, demanding them from his subordinates. In fact, his fanaticism for exactness makes him seem almost tyrannical. He wishes no one to meddle with his work or ideas. Being a strong and positive soul, he naturally has more enemies than friends. Such friends as he has are very sincere, however, and admire him for his exactitude.

Number three is the key note to his experiences in this incarnation. This means a very creative imagination, highly attuned nervous organism. Many changes and much travel. Much change during the first three years of his young life. During fourth year, the soul made a definite stand in order to accomplish what it came here to do. Up to twelve years of age he was under Karmic Law, hemmed in by environing circumstances, but at twelve the soul declares its freedom and has many experiences. At nineteen years of age a great change comes into operation. In February of 1892, a certain cycle was completed, bringing him into new surroundings and the determination to conquer. This is followed again by the meeting of an old Karmic Debt which certainly was paid and paid in full.

Then comes a period of recognition by the White Brotherhood and initiation into Nature's secrets and their protective influence, but along comes a test on the sex plane and in February of 1912 a separating force involving someone of the opposite sex comes into his life. For the soul above it is a test in initiation and this test again brings a new determination to conquer and accomplish the task the soul came to fulfill.

This is again followed by recognition from the Higher Brothers and their protection for a certain number of years. However, next comes a greater test on the sex plane and in May of 1925 his enemies are busy planning his downfall.

From 1925 to 1927 he must face the test of losing everything he values most on the Physical Plane, for he comes into the Christ number of Service and Sorrow. However, it is only a Test and after his birthday, November 28, 1927, he will again come under the protective influence of the Great White Brotherhood. His soul has been chosen a very hard incarnation, as he is trying to force humanity into a Sixth Race Consciousness and so meets with experiences in his own life that are necessary for humanity at large, before they can come into the greater Consciousness of the Sixth Race.

Brave soul! He has many separating forces tearing him into pieces, but he shall accomplish and his compensation will come in the end.

He has to transmute base metal into Gold, not only for himself but for humanity at large — a Jupiterian who has come here as a Messenger and is reaping what all advanced souls must reap in this benighted world.

Local Planets were not only circumspect about practicing Spectro-Chrome in the wake of all the legal action taken again practitioners but also that practitioners abide by the principles of their chapters. The First Milwaukee Wisconsin Planet, for instance, held a meeting on February 6, 1941, and the deputy officer, Frank S. Burns, warned the group that they must strictly adhere to their Constitution and Rules. He said "these are very trying times" and that no one should do anything that could "jeopardize Spectro-Chrome". He urged that if any affiliates were tonating sufferers but lacked the proper credentials to do so that they must stop treatment immediately.

Affiliates were asked to respond, and Emma Schroeder, the recorder, spoke up showcasing the fervor and ardor for Spectro-Chrome embraced by its users. She replied that:

no doubt every affiliate ... would like to see Spectro-Chrome prosper and progress to the ends of the Earth. When we consider medical science is in existence 6,000 years and our science only 21 years, it made good progress despite the odds. However, this does not mean that we must rest on our laurels. There is much work to be done.

In the Orange 1941 issue of *Spectro-Chrome*, Dinshah got a plum endorsement from a local journalist about what he was up against in America. The article was entitled "One Man Against an Unholy Alliance Battling for the Benefit of Mankind" and it was written by Shike Levine, the editor of the Bridgeton, New Jersey *Record*. Here is Levine's article as it appeared in *Spectro-Chrome*:

> Were the Medical Trust the only foe of Colonel Dinshah P. Ghadiali and Spectro-Chrome, his achievements would be classed as amazing. But to add to the American Medical Association such noted opposition as the powerful Liquor, Meat, Drug and Tobacco interests, one must look with awe at the success of one man who single-handed has been a match for such a ruthless combine.

This selfish combine controls the organs of publicity: radio, newspapers and magazines. Through such control, they have been able to foist their mercenary principles upon an innocent public and prevent the people from learning the facts about Spectro-Chrome.

This action by the unholy alliance is understandable. If the people were informed of Spectro-Chrome and subscribed to the great benefits resulting from adherence to its philosophy, the people would no longer go to medical doctors, would discontinue drinking liquor, stop eating meat, quit smoking and chewing tobacco and love without drugs and medicine, as well as destructive surgery.

Such condition would mean the end of the selfish quintet and it would mean the end of millionaires who obtained their wealth from stuffing the public with their injurious products.

Some day, the majority of people will learn of the unselfish fight Colonel Dinshah and Spectro-Chrome have been waging for the benefit of mankind and some day the nation will revere and honor the one man who battled such great odds to bring a new Health Science to the people.

Testimonials continued to pour into the Spectro-Chrome Institute from satisfied users of the healing art. Here is a letter from Greta R., of Scarsdale, New York, as reproduced in the June (Turquoise) 1941 issue of *Spectro-Chrome*:

A few months ago I was in a terrible accident, severing my nose in two. I began to tonate with your Spectro-Chrome and healed a terribly disfigured face in three weeks without even stitching it into place. Medical doctors thought me crazy when I said I could heal it with Spectro-Chrome. I returned to my place of business after four days of tonation. The terrible shock my nervous system got in the crash responded well to Turquoise.

Many of my friends do not believe Spectro-Chrome did the work, but what can I do when I already have it proven that it did!

Also from the same issue:

I am improving so nicely that my neighbors are amazed. I have lived in this neighborhood for 19 years and doctored all the time, but could not get better. Since I have Spectro-Chrome I do not have to see a doctor. Thank God for that and for Spectro-Chrome. The son of George F. came to my home here to collect on my coal bill and he asked me what I was doing for myself, as he never knew me to look so well. I told him I had a Spectro-Chrome and no more doctors for me. He said his father has been in poor health for years, could not get any thing to do him any good; he was going to have his father get a Spectro-Chrome right away; he thought it would help him. The next day his father came and I sent the order for him. *Submitted by Ida M. G., St. Louis, Missouri.*

My disorder called "Chronic disease of the spinal cord" came to my notice in 1929. I had very much pain in my leg and was treated for rheumatism at that time with no result. I got steadily worse and it afflicted the whole left side of my body. Leg, hip, stomach, arm and hand. I had to give up my work. I am walking with cane ever since. No medical doctor or hospital gave me relief. I went to a hospital for twelve weeks for observation and observation on the spine "to renew the spinal fluid". I had this done four times in four years. No result.

I started with Spectro-Chrome in 1938. I had better results from it after stopping all medicine and put on the Rational Food of Man. My digestion is much better and elimination regular. Pain in my right shoulder which I suffered for years is almost all gone. *Submitted by Otto F., Bridgeton, New Jersey.*

22

DINSHAH CONTINUES HIS SPECTRO-CHROME BUSINESS

Spectro-Chrome affiliates in Portland, the place where Dinshah's arrest years earlier led to his incarceration in a federal penitentiary, requested information on how to form a Planet branch in their city, as well as, if possible, a visit from Dinshah himself. Dinshah responded by saying he would come. He loaded his 1941 Plymouth truck with his healing therapy science apparatus. On June 14, 1941 Dinshah left his home in Malaga, New Jersey, and drove alone across the country. He kept a journal of his trip and thought it would "show to anyone doubting the value of the Rational Food of Man, what a man of 67, weighing only 120 pounds, can do on a single, simple meal a day, with a light breakfast and nothing else." When it came time to sleep, Dinshah parked in "Auto Courts", staying in a hotel only once, and, he wrote, "all the way through even cooked his own vegetarian meals."

Dinshah arrived in Portland on Sunday evening at 6 o'clock on June 22, 1941. He was to give free lectures for five nights at the Masonic Temple starting on Saturday evening, June 28. While he was setting up his equipment in the Masonic Temple's De Molay Room, Oregon State Police detective Alvin Rea and Russell Bly of the Better Business Bureau entered the room and inquired about his activities. Dinshah took them to his motel room beyond the city limits to show him his credentials, of which he had brought a large supply, and from there they went to the police station where a sergeant inquired further of his activities. Dinshah then left.

Dinshah soon presented a series of lectures about Spectro-Chrome Metry, his Rational Food of Man diet, alcohol and tobacco, his life history, and rules of Spectro-Chrome Metrists. He showed slides and motion pictures of his Spectro-Chrome Institute that provided details of its operation. On each of the first two nights some 225 affiliates and non-affiliates attended. Numerous testimonials were given, with affiliates telling how sufferers they treated were successfully normalated when conventional medical doctors could not help them. Detective Rea and Mr. Bly attended one of the lectures, and hearing the satisfaction of affiliates who had purchased Spectro-Chrome equipment, spoke graciously to Dinshah as they left the lecture.

On July 13, 1941, Dinshah returned home and started working at his institute again. But he knew he had to change the structure of his operation lest he be driven out of business. As he noted in the September (Violet) 1941 issue of *Spectro-Chrome*, he had formed his Spectro-Chrome Institute in 1920 as a proprietary entity and less than two years later converted it into a corporation of business stock. It wasn't until 1926 that he really began selling stock owing to his expensive legal battles that he felt were instigated by the American Medical Association. The financial burden of legal expenses was then compounded by the tax burdens of the New Deal that small corporations like his had difficulty surviving. So he moved for a dissolution of the Spectro-Chrome Institute (paying the preferred stockholders at his own expense); this took place on September 15, 1941.

Under a new corporation, Dinshah described his entity as follows:

Dinshah Spectro-Chrome Institute is a totally closed organization. It creates no sales and deals solely with those who are affiliated with it. It grants a Benefit Studentship for $90.00 and presents to the Student a Spectro-Chrome Home Guide, a complete Spectro-Chrome Equipment for exemplification of the Science, Free Guidance during life of the Affiliate, for all persons in immediate family of the Benefit Student, Free Spectro-Chrome and Favorscope for the current year, Free Benefit Meetings, besides numerous advantages and Auxiliary Benefits. No profit is intended and all the proceeds go to the advancement of Spectro-Chrome Metry. The annual fees and dues thereafter are only $3.00 for maintaining the Benefit Affiliation. Thus, for less than 1 cent a day, all that the medical doctors, surgeons and their odoriferous hospitals could offer, is brought in the true Godly form to the family home, for better health, better education, better science, better service and better brotherhood ...

Meanwhile, the affiliates of the Planets around the country continued to profess their belief in the effectiveness of Spectro-Chrome based on their personal experience with it and were for the most part adamant that they were not pawns of a quack. At the First Milwaukee, Wisconsin meeting held at the Hotel Wisconsin on February 6, 1941, the Deputy officer, Frank S. Burns, asserted he was not in the "sucker" class of people who get taken in by quacks. He said he had had a physical problem and had gone to several different healers for relief but no one had helped. Then someone mentioned Spectro-Chrome and he did not look into it until months later when a relative brought it up. He researched how to buy a machine, eventually did, and was very happy with the relief it brought him.

Dinshah was always promoting the simplicity of using Spectro-Chrome, which of course inferred that because anyone could learn to use it, it largely removed the need for medical doctors. In one issue of *Spectro-Chrome* he wrote "How even housewives in remote parts of the country are using Spectro-Chrome with success" and then quoted a letter from Josie of Oregon who wrote how she came down with the flu but "got over it in 36 hours thanks to Spectro-Chrome." She then told the story of how she had four teeth extracted and experienced hemorrhaging. The dentist said he had to leave his office but would return soon to address it. She responded "No, I have a light that will take care of it." The dentist walked away in disgust but when she returned the next morning he was astonished by how her mouth looked, saying it looked like the extraction took place a week ago. "Yes," she beamed to the dentist, "I can do in two hours with Spectro-Chrome what it will take an entire week to accomplish." His curiosity piqued, the dentist said he now had to visit Josie at home to take a look at her Spectro-Chrome machine for himself.

Not all letters received by Dinshah and his Spectro-Chrome Institute were positive and the originator of the colored-light therapy wasn't abashed about printing the negative ones in *Spectro-Chrome*, too. For instance, while he often received requests from affiliates to send literature to family members and friends, it was his policy not to unless someone personally requested it. But a newspaper editor sent him a list of people and, making a rare exception to his policy, Dinshah dispatched literature to the people on the editor's list. One of the recipients, Harold H. Beebe of Pitman, New Jersey, wrote back saying:

> Kindly be advised that I do not now have, nor at any time ever did have any interest whatsoever in your Spectro-Chrome cure-all or publication. Neither am I curious concerning your insidious philosophy ... by whom our American government is operated.
>
> If your publication expects to disseminate propaganda detrimental to the President of the United States, the ladies and gentlemen of the Congress of the United States, or of the people of the United States, it has missed its aim badly in my case.
>
> If you are not satisfied with our government as it is presently constituted, you are invited and certainly privileged to go back to wherever you came from—and make it snappy.

Further literature from you will positively not be accepted by this house.

Dinshah wrote Pitman back saying his name had been submitted by a newspaper editor and copies of *Spectro-Chrome* were sent to him even though it was against the Institute's strict rule not to send literature to anyone who didn't request it. Then he added:

I am quite able to answer every uncalled, offensive and insulting paragraph in your letter, but, thinking it beneath my dignity as a scientific researcher and an editor, I am printing your letter verbatim, in my Spectro-Chrome, leaving it to my intelligent readers to answer you.

There was Albert Hale, a normalator from Plymouth Wisconsin, who told about a woman from Sheboygan who suffered from painful post-partum swelling, or what he called "milk leg". She also got headaches and her other leg swelled up, and wasn't happy with the results she obtained from Spectro-Chrome so she went back to her medical doctor. It turned out that after seeking help from her doctor her condition worsened so she went back to Spectro-Chrome. She wasn't sleeping well and having read of the wonderful results people obtain with Spectro-Chrome in the magazines and not obtaining similar results she was becoming discouraged again. Hale asked Dinshah for advice.

"Even I have to die," Dinshah responded. "Milk leg is worse than varicose veins. I never claimed that Spectro-Chrome is a 'cure-all'. All that I ever claimed for it is that it is capable of doing what drugs and medicine can do and much that they cannot do. With the proper food, mental attitude and so forth, Spectro-Chrome will give proper service. This is a similar case of making a rooster lay eggs. Similar also to phthisis. Seal the cavity so there is no more hemorrhage; but I cannot grow a new ovary where there is none."

Hale later reported that the woman emitted some large chunks of blood and her headaches were relived.

Dinshah avidly continued publishing his *Spectro-Chrome* magazine, attending annual conventions of Spectro-Chrome Metrists, speaking at Planet meetings around the country and giving Spectro-Chrome courses, but for all his hope and ambition to get Spectro-Chrome in every American home, he must have been harboring doubts about his healing system's future by the mid-1940s. Federal agents around the country were invading the homes of owners of Spectro-Chrome machines and confiscating the equipment. Although the government acknowledged that at the very worst these machines were harmless, and despite the owners' strenuous objections, the agents seized the machines and destroyed them. Much publicity and fanfare accompanied these raids and newspapers printed pictures showing the destruction of this "fake" equipment. The U.S. Post Office Department issued a Fraud Order prohibiting Dinshah from receiving mail and returned all correspondence to him to the senders.

Dinshah conducted his Institute with full transparency. He noted in the April (Lemon) 1942 issue of *Spectro-Chrome* that when he changed his organization's status from a manufacturing business to a non-profit corporation many affiliates could not understand how an international body could be "totally independent and exist without accepting outside financial support." But he said the key to Spectro-Chrome's survival was "unselfish support". He then told of the more than two decades of indefatigable work he had put into his healing system and that he never accepted graft of any kind. At the end of his discussion he listed the Spectro-Chrome Institute's final income tax report for 1941. Among the figures listed for receipts were the Institute's gross sales of $44,714.71, rents of $435, discounts earned of $18, and "refund from Treasury Department for taxes illegally collected" of $827.42. Disbursements included merchandise bought for furniture (less material previous year's purchase) coming to $17,024.44, salaries and labor for $7,536, commissions to independent field solicitors for $45,794, taxes of $2,160.21, heat and light amounting to $1,298.88, repairs for $594.21, and legal fees of $556.86. The total gross income of $45,995.13 less the disbursements of $41,333.93 left a net income of $4,661.20. But Dinshah protested it was not really the institute's net income since it went to pay previous years' losses and obligations for which the Treasury Department in recent years had stopped allowing deductions. He noted "the Originator still works for the Corporation without salary and so does his wife, all the children, seven in number, assisting their parents in the unique service. There is a private school maintained on the premises for the education of the youngsters and each in his after-study hours takes pride in doing something to help the Cause."

23

THE U.S. POST OFFICE DEPARTMENT GOES AFTER DINSHAH

Dinshah would usually get wind of the latest trouble brewing his way either by personal visits from legal authorities or by the U.S. mail. Sometimes his Spectro-Chrome students would inform him of the latest flap blowing his way but usually it came in the form of a detective or a stamped envelope. The latter form was the vehicle of choice for delivery of the latest bad news for him.

A letter arrived at the Spectro-Chrome Institute on August 21, 1942 naming several people and entities (such as the Spectro-Chrome Institute) as "engaged in conducting a scheme or device for obtaining money through the mails by means of false or fraudulent pretenses, representation or promises", which violated postal laws of the United States, specifically sections 259 and 732 of Title 39 of the U.S. Code. Any person or entity found operating in violation of the statute could result in the Postmaster General withholding their mail and stopping payment of any U.S. money orders to them. Since a major part of the Spectro-Chrome Institute's business endeavors was mailing its magazine and literature and cashing money orders people sent to them, this latest letter threatened to severely hamper the enterprise.

A hearing was held on September 21, 1942 in Washington, D.C. to determine why the U.S. Post Office should not withhold delivery of mail and money orders to the Spectro-Chrome Institute and Dinshah. He did not attend the hearing since he had responded to the original letter with a package of supporting materials that he hoped would result in the case being dropped. From the testimony at the hearing it turned out that the case spawned from complaints from a disgruntled Spectro-Chrome user and the brother-in-law of a disgruntled Spectro-Chrome user. Consequently, a Post Office Inspector named Karl M. Foust had investigated the background of Dinshah and his Spectro-Chrome Institute, and subsequently enrolled as a Benefit Student in Dinsah's Institute under the fake name of Amelia Regina Wylie of Ridgeway, Missouri. Foust appeared as a witness along with physicians and a scientist who all denounced Spectro-Chrome as having no therapeutic value whatsoever.

A transcript of 85 pages of the hearing was sent to Dinshah, who received it on October 7, 1942. After being granted a few extensions to respond, Dinshah returned 60 pages of comments refuting statements given under oath. One by one he tore down the testimonies and called the physicist, who was on the AMA's Council of Physical Therapy, a "henchman of the American Medical Association".

In response to one New York physician who had gone to medical school in Hungary and called Dinshah's science a "complete system of fooling", Dinshah offered affidavits from Spectro-Chrome users proclaiming "Diabetes was normalated without insulin and without the stopping of starches and sugars, paralytics were made to walk, restored dying consumptives to health, eye disorders were normalated, cancer was controlled, tumors were normalated, arthritis was overcome, new skin was built in large areas."

Dinshah estimated that some 8,000 Spectro-Chrome machines were in use around the country treating as many as 25,000 people. "I had the honor to train in Spectro-Chrome Metry, hundreds of licensed medical doctors, surgeons, osteopathic physicians, dental surgeons and the like in 95 classes within 22 years," Dinshah wrote, "and I respectfully submit a few of their testimonials for your kind consideration. These testimonials were given by those doctors, not only after taking my course, but each of them used my Spectro-Chrome in daily practice."

A Fraud Order was issued by Frank C. Walker, the Postmaster General of the U.S. Post Office Department on December 22, 1942, forbidding the payment of any money order to Dinshah, the Spectro-Chrome Institute or any of the other individuals or entitles named on the initial Notice charging the parties with "conducting a scheme or device for obtaining money through the mails by means of false and fraudulent pretenses, representation and promises in violation of specified section of Title 39 of the U.S. Code"; as well as instructions for post offices to "return all letters, whether registered or not, and other mail matter which shall arrive at your office directed to the said concerns and parties to the postmasters at the offices at which they were originally mailed, to be delivered to the senders thereof, with the words 'Fraudulent: mail to this addressed returned by order of the Postmaster General'."

Dinshah responded to Postmaster General Frank Walker in a letter dated December 30, 1942. He refuted the charge that he and his Institute were "scheming for money" saying "We are a non-stock, non-profit corporation ... and *all* our activities and resources are centered in benefiting the ailing through our science of Spectro-Chrome unselfishly" and that "The service to our affiliates is available absolutely free and without any charge."

Dinshah submitted five case histories of sufferers giving their full names and stating that the Fraud Order could cause "potential death to some of these sufferers". He asked the Postmaster General to "modify your Fraud Order so as not to punish the innocent sick and suffering, thousands of whom are at present *exclusively* under our care and *free guidance*."

Pursuant to the Fraud Order, all mail delivery to the Spectro-

Chrome Institute was discontinued. The only way for anyone on the outside to reach anyone at the Institute was by telephone, telegraph or Railway Express. The termination of mail notwithstanding, Dinshah pledged to continue providing health services and free advice.

In a letter dated January 5, 1943, Vincent M. Miles in the Post Office Department's Office of the Solicitor wrote Dinshah that

> The evidence of this case clearly showed that the mails were being used in the operation of a scheme to defraud and in view thereof this office would not be warranted in recommending modification of the fraud order to permit resumption of operation of any part of the fraudulent enterprise, as requested by you.

Dinshah replied with a letter dated January 16, 1943. Vincent Miles promptly wrote Dinshah that since re-examination of the matter had shown that the Fraud Order was issued on the basis of overwhelming evidence, and that Dinshah had failed to show up at the hearing at his own option or present the testimony of any witnesses,

> revocation of the said fraud order to permit resumption of the fraudulent scheme formerly conducted by you through the mails is not warranted at this time.

So dedicated were Dinshah's followers that affiliates at the 23rd Annual Convention of Spectro-Chrome Metrists in Milwaukee pledged to raise money for a "Fraud Order Revocation" fund. Contributors were directed not to use the mail but send in contributions by Railway Express Agency and to make the donations payable to "Fraud Order Revocation Contribution".

At the 23rd Annual Convention the attendees passed a resolution to secure the help in the Fraud Order matter from Wisconsin Senator Robert La Follette, Jr. A letter dated January 11, 1943 and signed by

300 affiliates and Dinshah himself, was sent to the senator stating the charges made by the Postmaster General were false, that Spectro-Chrome was not a fraud, and, with the enclosure of a testimonial from former Milwaukee Mayor Daniel W. Hoan, who had purchased Spectro-Chrome equipment and once spoken at an Annual Convention, and asked that he "avail yourself of the evidence in this case and examine it, and we are sure you will find the charges unfounded."

In his affidavit, Hoan stated that he purchased Spectro-Chrome equipment for the use of him and his family and had "found it very helpful for many purposes beneficial to health and is still using the same," and that he "is personally acquainted with a great majority of the people who have attended the Colonel's lectures and courses and knows that they are well satisfied with the results that have been obtained from this system of Spectro-Chrome Metry."

Dinshah followed up the letter from the Annual Convention affiliates with letters from himself to Senator La Follette. In one, he wrote:

> Your illustrious father exposed extensive frauds in the Post Office Department in the time of President William McKinley; we look to you, his fearless and progressive son for help in saving our humanitarian, scientific activities from destruction from the machinations of the medical lobby which has caused the Post Office Department against us in a fraudulent way.

Dinshah's next move was to file a bill of complaint against the Postmaster General and Assistant Postmaster of Malaga, New Jersey alleging "unfair, unjust treatment and charges perjury and forgery were used to frame him and his corporation." He also filed a petition with the District Court for the State of New Jersey for a temporary restraining order and injunction against the Fraud Order. On February 26, 1943, Dinshah filed a brief with the District Court for the District of New Jersey in which he affirmed such items as that no fraud had been created, no promises had been made about cures, his use of the mail was not fraudulent, no false statements had been made, and Spectro-Chrome had been proven to be beneficial.

Meanwhile, contributions for the Fraud Order Revocation were starting to pour in. Before long over 300 donations were received, and Dinshah printed the full names of the contributors in his *Spectro-Chrome* magazine. The U.S. Government filed a "Memo of Law" in the New Jersey District Court requesting Dinshah's application for a restraining order should be dismissed, which Dinshah quickly responded.

On July 9, 1943 Judge John Davis of the U.S. District Court in Camden, New Jersey entered an opinion for the court that it did not have jurisdiction to dismiss the petition for temporary restraint of the Fraud Order. Subsequently, on August 9, 1943, Dinshah wrote the Post Office Department that he wished to petition the Post Office Department for a "reopening and rehearing" of his Fraud Order. In response, he was requested to supply "alleged specific errors" in order for the case to be reopened. Dinshah did and was requested to the Office of the Solicitor on October 15, 1943. Dinshah requested "inasmuch as your Post Office Department has the power and authority to call witnesses in such investigation," that certain witnesses whose names followed be summoned to appear at the hearing, and he enclosed a certified check for $1,000 to cover their expenses. The request was denied and Dinshah's check was returned. Subsequent appeals by Dinshah over the next couple years to have these witnesses appear were likewise denied and a trial date was set for January 8, 1945.

Through a mutual friend Dinshah met a man named John Crim, who was said to be influential in Washington's political circles. Crim arranged for a rehearing which occurred on May 2, 1945. Fifteen witnesses came in Dinshah's behalf from as far away as Detroit, Milwaukee and St. Louis. However, the Assistant Solicitor ordered the court reporter to leave. Dinshah protested and was informed a recording machine would make the record of the proceedings. The

Assistant Solicitor then announced that the only witnesses that would be allowed would be "expert medical testimony". The witnesses that came for Dinshah were Spectro-Chrome users who wanted to testify how much the healing art had helped them recover from illness.

On August 29, 1945 U.S Attorney Thorn Lord notified Dinshah that a grand jury indicted him on five counts for "using the mails in a scheme to defraud". Dinshah subsequently appeared at the U.S. District Court in Camden and pleaded not guilty. A conviction could result in a five-year jail sentence and a fine of $1,000. Dinshah was released without bail. The case dragged on until eventually at trial the Fraud Order stayed in place and Dinshah was fined $1,000 but did not have to serve jail time.

24

SPECTRO-CHROME AND THE ST. LOUIS BETTER BUSINESS BUREAU

On March 25, 1943, Kenneth W. Hood, the manager of the Merchandising Division of the Better Business Bureau located in the Arcadia Building in St. Louis sent off a letter to Clemens Neumann, a Spectro-Chrome therapist in the city. He wrote that the Better Business Bureau had become aware that Neumann was "treating people by means of the so-called 'Spectro-Chrome Therapy' ... originated by one Dinshah P. Ghadiali" and asked if he was "aware that his man has been condemned as a quack by the American Medical Association with a record of his convictions for law violations?" Hood asked Neumann if he could give the Bureau "a good reason why we should not warn the public against the methods you are using."

Neumann wrote Hood back on April 7, 1943 saying:

Before I answer your inquiry it will be necessary for me to know first-hand from you what information the American Medical Association and you have about this man.

Hood immediately wrote back requesting Neumann to call him to let him know when he could come to his office, at which time he would "be given the opportunity to read what the American Medical Association wrote about Dinshah P. Ghadiali.

Neumann replied:

> If you have nothing to give me in writing or print about what you may have to say, I have no reason to visit your office or involve myself in other people's affairs.

This response seemed to have exasperated Hood as on May 6, 1943 he wrote to Neumann:

> It is your privilege to do as you please about visiting our office and reading the material published by the American Medical Association about Dinshah P. Ghadiali. In the future, do not forget that we offered you the opportunity.
>
> We should think that you would be interested from your own standpoint in finding what you could inasmuch as you apparently are risking the good health of some members of the public through your use of this machine. In fact, we have the name and address of one party who attributes the death of a member of the family to reliance on you and his machine treatments instead of consulting with a doctor.

With his own success in using Spectro-Chrome, Neumann was a staunch defender of Dinshah's healing art. On May 25, 1943 he wrote Hood back:

> I received your letter of May 6, 1943 and thank you for the unusual interest in my welfare! However, I may state that I know Colonel Dinshah and his work more than you ever will know because I have been affiliated with his Organization for over ten

years. I feel you could not tell me anything more about the man and his activities than I know myself.

Since Spectro-Chrome started in 1920, the fight of the American Medical Association to down the man and his system are well known. I am acquainted with the inside facts. I send you a copy of the libel of the A.M.A. of January 1924, Exhibit A. Dinshah openly answered it fully in his *Spectro-Chrome* magazine ... Exhibit B.

That being unanswered and more dirt being thrown against him, he sent an open Challenge against the A.M.A. and the Chicago Better Business Bureau as published in *Spectro-Chrome*, September 1934, Exhibit C.

In Buffalo, New York, the Better Business Bureau was instrumental in dragging Dinshah through the Erie County Medical Society, in the Supreme Court there, and Exhibit D will show you how the man received an acquittal. In that case, in the Supreme Court much was openly stated about the Better Business Bureau. The complainant himself is on record as calling it "the bastard government". The last three lines in your letter are absurd because the medical doctors do not save 100 in a hundred.

I give no service to the public and my services are exclusively extended to Affiliates of the Organization, who mostly join us after having one foot in the grave because of some wrong treatment by medical doctors.

If you know anything more than I do about Dinshah and his work you may freely send it to me and I promise you careful attention.

There was no immediate response from the Better Business Bureau to Neumann's letter, and Dinshah surmised that the Bureau huddled with the A.M.A., which as an organization proclaiming a monopoly on the healing art the U.S. Supreme Court had on January 18, 1943 declared guilty of conspiracy to restrain trade and fined

$2,500, in planning its next step. Sure enough, an article titled "Hocus-Pocus?" appeared on the front page of the July 8, 1943 issue of the *St. Louis Better Business Bureau Bulletin*:

Cures for human ailments in the shape of a magic machine are offered to St. Louisans under the very scientific-sounding name of "Spectro-Chrome Therapy". This system of treatment, which involves the use of "attuned color waves" on a definite time schedule, is the brainchild of one Dinshah P. Ghadiali, a Hindu, whom the American Medical Association has condemned as a quack. The Bureau has the name of one woman who attributes the death of her husband to misplaced faith in this machine and system of treatment.

Dinshah himself responded to Hood saying "Hocus Pocus?" was "an unwarranted and unjustified article libeling me and my Science of Spectro-Chrome." He chastised Hood for printing the article without an investigation and denied he was either a Hindu or quack. Dinshah printed all the correspondence between Hood and Neumann in *Spectro-Chrome* and enclosed copies of the magazine with his letter to Hood. He asked Hood to do the same to print the correspondence in the *Better Business Bureau Bulletin* (Dinshah referred to it in his letter as a "scandal sheet") and challenged Hood to "accept my challenge to expose me before the public or meet me on the open debating platform when I am next in your city of St Louis, which will not be long." Dinshah offered Hood the opportunity to have any reply to his letter printed in Spectro-Chrome "without any censorship to give my readers your side of the story" and concluded by defiantly stating "If you have American Red Blood in your arteries better than the American Blood I have, you should not hesitate to put the whole issue before the public or apologize as a man for your cowardly attack."

Despite his strong words, Dinshah indubitably had no animosity toward Hood. As Dinshah once wrote:

We bear no malice or ill feeling even towards our worst opponents.

We shall leave them to their own reactions, so wisely regulated by the Grand Architect of the Universe, through the immutable Laws of Karma recognized as the Laws of Retributive Justice: may they get good sense to read the Handwriting on The Wall!

Hood never replied to Dinshah's open challenge.

25

THE SPECTO-CHROME INSTITUTE FIRE

Tuesday, January 2, 1945 was a bright, clear day in southern New Jersey, with strong winds whipping the frigid air. It was just the second day of the new year, but it was business as usual at the 23-acre Spectro-Chrome Institute on West Boulevard in Malaga.

Dinshah was in his office in the large main building of the Institute talking with a married couple from Yeadon, Pennsylvania. The husband wanted to become a Benefit Student so he could tonate his wife who was ill, and Dinshah was inquiring about her condition. After an interview, Dinshah requested his son Darius to go get a machine for the couple.

Sometime before 10 a.m., as Dinshah was consulting with the visting couple, his son Jal suddenly burst into the office to say smoke was coming from the eave of the south side of the two-and-a-half-story, 30-room building. The building housed the Institute's laboratory, auditorium, school, and living quarters where Dinshah and his family resided.

There had been a devastating fire in the area just a couple days before, in Glassboro, about ten miles to the north. One of the city's major historic buildings had been razed in the blaze so the possibility of a fire at the Institute was something on the minds of its occupants.

Dinshah, 71 years old, ran outside to assess the situation. Only a small amount of smoke was visible and no flames could be seen. Roshan went to the garage housing the Institute's fire engine and pulled out its hose. Darius grabbed it and aimed it at the eave while Roshan activated the soda/acid tanks, but apparently not enough pressure was generated and consequently very little water came out. Their brothers Cyrus and Sarosh all rushed over to see if they could help put out the small fire. Dinshah then ran inside the building to call the local fire department, and very shortly an engine arrived.

With high winds blowing the fire was spreading quickly through the framed structure. It now looked like the fire was going to cause much damage to the property, and Dinshah rushed in to retrieve important legal papers. Meanwhile, the fire was starting to rage and as the firemen were battling it from their truck Irene quickly gathered all her boys outside and away from the blistering building. At the same time, Dinshah, who had stepped out of the building after grabbing his legal papers, realized there were many other vital documents and affidavits he needed as well as money orders totaling thousands of dollars and rushed back in but was blinded by black smoke and had to retreat, lest he be consumed by it. But he did manage to make it to the basement where he turned off the electrical switches located in the heating plants.

The fire was so out of control that several local fire departments were called in and state police officers sped to the Institute also. Soon, firemen of about a half-dozen fire companies were fighting to contain the flames. Parts of the building were already succumbing to the flames so the firefighters put their efforts into sections they thought they could save.

People were pouring onto the property now. Neighbors from far and near, people passing through the area, newspaper reporters all gathered to watch the fire ravage the Institute. State police officers kept the spectators at bay.

Parts of the building started to crumble, and with them valuable materials related to Spectro-Chrome were destroyed. Machines, slides, apparati, equipment, books, files, documents, personal records, newspaper articles about him — virtually everything Dinshah had built, accumulated and saved from his professional career was ravaged. Of course, desks, chairs, telephones, and other office equipment were likewise destroyed as well as family belongings including all their clothing and personal treasures.

As other buildings on the property appeared ready to be consumed by flames, the firemen turned their hoses where the flames were roaring. Windows broke, machines were ruined and water covered the floors. The damage to the Institute amounted to about $100,000.

A few hours after the fire had started, the engine companies began leaving the premises. The main building was entirely destroyed with hot cinders remaining in the rubble and Malaga firemen stayed behind to make sure they didn't blow into the nearby thickets.

Local newspapers ran articles about the fire the next day. But one of the papers, the *Philadelphia Record*, instead of objectively reporting the devastating event, managed to be cynical in its coverage. Running under the headline "Blaze Destroys Institute of Scion of Fire Worshippers," the article stated Dinshah Ghadiali claimed to be a "descendant of the fire worshippers of ancient Persia" and went on to say that after the fire broke out "One might have expected Ghadiali to whip into an intricate scimitar dance, uttering incantations to the fire gods." The article mentioned that Dinshah had run for governor of New Jersey in 1937 but that "The State never got around to counting the number (if any) of Parsee votes he corralled."

The fire was reported by a newspaper as being of "unknown origin" but Dinshah's family attributed it to a sooty boiler recently installed to heat the eastern part of the building where the flue was connected to a small unlined brick chimney (later reports of an airplane reportedly heard overhead about one half hour before the fire was discovered and suspected to have dropped an incendiary bomb were dismissed by the Dinshah family as being completely rubbish).

Whatever its origin, the fire that started on a typical day and within a short time span of less than two hours consumed a lifetime of work was but the latest setback to Dinshah. Legal actions were looming over his professional pursuits at the same time as Spectro-Chrome affiliates all over the country depended on his guidance and leadership. But while the fire was devastating to his Institute, no member of his family was hurt and he took it with his usual equanimity in the face of trouble. As was written about Dinshah in *Spectro-Chrome*:

He thought of the glory of the Lord Zoroaster who was murdered by a stab in the back. He thought of the great Lord Jesus the Christ who was crucified because he did not conform to the viewpoints of his thoughtless opponents. Dinshah is only a servant of the world which is imbued in a turmoil of greed, selfishness and materialism. He left the land of his birth and became a citizen of the United States of America because of the reverence in which he held the glorious Constitution of this Country. What this Country gave him in return is well known to his affiliates and is recorded in the ethers of history.

Dinshah, the humble servant of suffering humanity is down but *not out*, because *truth* may be temporarily defeated, but can *never be conquered*.

26

THE 1945 AND 1946 FDA TRIALS

The U.S. Food and Drug Administration went after Spectro-Chrome and Dinshah twice in the mid-1940s. The first trial at the United States District Court, Eastern District of New York was held in Brooklyn with District Judge Robert A. Inch presiding and Assistant U.S. Attorney Morris K. Siegel appearing for the government. The trial began on May 14, 1945 and ended on June 26, 1945. The government charged Dinshah with making "false and misleading statements". The U.S. government called 40 witnesses and Dinshah called 111 witnesses, but this time Dinshah's witnesses were not medical doctors such as Kate Baldwin or Welcome A. Hanor who had testified for him before since they were no longer living. Dinshah's witnesses were now Spectro-Chrome users who could only offer their unverified successes with his system. The government, on the other hand, brought in scientists and physicians including a Nobel Prize-winning physicist, an astrophysicist-secretary of the Smithsonian Institution, and Dr. Morris Fishbein, the AMA *Journal* editor, and was able to convince the jury of twelve women that Spectro-Chrome could be harmful. The physicians who testified expressed their belief that the labeling on Spectro-Chrome literature would prevent an ill person from seeking their help and was therefore "dangerous to public health". Dinshah was fined $2,531.85 and "enjoined and restrained from directly or indirectly causing the introduction or delivery for introduction into interstate commerce ... of any article or device ... labeled similarly to the device herein condemned ... or which carries literature bearing a ... resemblance to the label or literature of this cause."

The U.S. government was relentless in its pursuit of Dinshah and Spectro-Chrome. On October 21, 1946 Dinshah P. Ghadiali and the Dinshah Spectro-Chrome Institute were tried in the United States District Court for the District of New Jersey for an indictment with twelve counts. The defendants were charged with engaging in interstate commerce of twelve devices on which their labeling contained "false and misleading statements". The trial commenced on October 21, 1946. Dinshah represented both himself and the Institute before Judge Philip Forman.

The government claimed that Dinshah's and his Institute's Spectro-Chrome machines, which were shipped in interstate commerce, did not have any therapeutic value and were therefore misleading in relation to Section 502 (a) of the Federal Food, Drug and Cosmetic Act.

The trial was held and the jury, essentially composed of twelve housewives, delivered its verdict on January 7, 1947. Dinshah and the Dinshah Spectro-Chrome Institute were found guilty on all counts as charged. The surgeon Dr. Kate Baldwin, if she had been alive, might have appeared as a witness on behalf of Dinshah but unfortunately she had died in Lawrenceville, Pennsylvania on January 17, 1935. She was Spectro-Chrome's greatest medical doctor champion, and her death was a great loss for Dinshah.

With the guilty verdict a sentence was to be handed down. The opinion of the trial court on the sentence was given and its veiled racism, unqualified denigration of color-light healing and outrageous comparison of Dinshah to history's most evil dictator, among other disparaging comments, doubtlessly exasperated the man in question.

The trial court even denigrated the scores of Spectro-Chrome users who came from all over the county at their own expense to testify on Dinshah's behalf by saying that the users had been hoodwinked. Here is an extract from the trial court:

Mr. Ghadiali, you express great admiration for America and your American citizenship but you have substantially rejected the custom and general mode of life in America. You have walled yourself up in distinctive dress, a failure generally to associate yourself with the people except in certain lines. This you have done not only to yourself but you have conceived it desirable to rear and raise your family in the same way but to this no one could complain in America, which is a country for different people to live in unitedly.

However, that very isolationism of yours is characteristic of a general pattern or design in your life, as it was laid open here in the many weeks of trial, a trial that I think was in all respects in the American tradition of fairness. You represented yourself as counsel, and as far as it was possible every facility was made available to you to exploit your defense to a jury of citizens so that final judgment upon the facts and the law could eventually be made upon the charges of the government.

Your mode of living followed a pattern or design where you were the central figure of government in the little world you created. You made your geographical settlement, you made your laws and you made your own government, and wherever this was consistent with the laws of the United States again no complaint could be made against you.

Then, many years ago, you hit upon an idea of an alleged system of healing people. It apparently consisted of a recommendation to follow a diet and of following prohibitory regulations against use of alcohol and tobacco, coupled with the distribution of a device designed to shine, as you alleged, beneficial attuned color waves upon the human body in order to cure its ills.

Of course the diet and the prohibitions against the use of alcohol and tobacco, I suppose, are nearly as old as man himself except that the use of tobacco is a more modern indulgence. These were nothing new. Such instructions may well have had some benefit.

However, along with your invention of the alleged beneficial waves of color you made rather cunning use of the New Jersey Corporation laws upon which you built the so-called Dinshah Spectro-Chrome Institute. And you would have me think that a wide chasm separates you, Dinshah P. Ghadiali, from the Spectro-Chrome Institute. This can be done with the corporate laws of our state in a technical sense, but, Mr. Ghadiali, I can only feel, and I think I am justified in feeling, that only the most fragile veil separates the individual Dinshah P. Ghadiali from the so-called corporate entity.

Other shrewd implementations were contrived by you to turn this entire matter of treating people for the sickness into a special group of fraternal brotherhood as you have sometimes called it yourself.

I conceive it now to be my duty to carry out that jury verdict, not with the idea of vindictiveness or retribution because that is not in the area of what one human being or a society of human beings should do to another human being, but very, very emphatically is it my duty to implement that decision of the jury so as bring to a stop the evil suggested in the verdict. There is evil in this thing. Whether it is by design upon your part I am not at all sure. I am inclined now to feel that if such ever existed now by some aberration of brain or mind you conceive yourself to be the creator of a small universe and to be the creator of a system of healing that is the greatest boon to mankind in the terminology or the equivalent thereof you describe yourself in your encyclopedia. I am convinced that by some form of self-hypnosis you are obsessed with the idea that you have been commissioned by God to bring your claimed only true art of healing to mankind.

In a case in which you had ample opportunity to bring forward any kind of evidence that would fit within the framework of our judicial system of admission of testimony you completely failed to bring any convincing proof of the value of this system of healing except as it came from the lips of 100 or so or 150 poor souls who, without any knowledge of the human body, either with illnesses or with the thought that they had illnesses, swore that they felt themselves relived by the use of the mechanism. This was very unimpressive, very unimpressive. Not a single scientist from all of those who are found in this country was brought forward to testify to the efficacy or the realism of any scientific principles which you invoked, and the court can only feel that these 112 witnesses whom you brought here, culled from the thousands who used the machine, were simply dupes of your suggestions and highly exaggerated imaginations.

There is an additional element of public danger to this business of delusion upon the part of those who parted with their $90 and perhaps more money that went into the pockets of these so-called normalators — and may I say that of those who appeared upon the stand certainly none was in the least qualified to minister to the ills of human beings, not the least, by fundamental education or experience. There is always the inherent danger that people with very dangerous ills existing in their inception who should have advantages of progressive medical treatment that is so well known that no one can ridicule or deride it, who will substitute your system until it is too late for them to be helped. Of course the medical cart is not perfect by any means. Many of its frontiers are still open, but people who are in the incipient stage of cancer or diabetes or many other illnesses may well fall victims to death by reason of being diverted from well-known practices in the medical profession to exposing themselves to the diet that you suggest and the shining on themselves of utterly meaningless colored lights.

Now, the matter of sentence is before me. As the government has indicated, a maximum of $24,000 in fines and a maximum of 12 years in prison for the individual defendant is possible.

I have given respectful consideration to the government's suggestion that imprisonment is in order in this case. Having in mind, as I said before, that the one purpose of the court should be to implement the verdict to the extent that the transgression against the law should be stopped once and for all, it may very well be that the government's suggestions of imprisonment may be the only effective way of doing it. My consideration of its recommendation, however, does not lead in that direction.

This is slanted first by the great age of the defendant who is now 73 years. Although he has expressed the notion that he might go on for another 73 years, and as far as I am concerned he may very well do so, I am afraid that would be in the area of prediction by that genuine or apocryphal Russian scientist recently reported in the press who said that we would all soon be living to 125 years and he died soon after he made the prediction at the tender age of 63 or 64.

Mr. Ghadiali, you are an old man. You may sit down.

Mr. Ghadiali: I thought your Honor wanted me to stand for sentence.

The Court: No. You know my dignity is not easily infringed upon.

Mr. Ghadiali: Thank you, sir.

The Court:

You are an old man. It does not seem necessary to me to so regulate your life so that you should perhaps die in prison, as there would be grave danger of your doing if I gave you an extended prison sentence. I am not thinking only of the matter in that field of emotion or sentiment. I am thinking of it in another matter. In the creation of this little universe of your own, like all of those who do that sort of thing, you have attracted a fringe around you. That has become quite a large number. To send you to prison would be to perhaps push that fringe over the ledge that it even now teeters on into becoming a cult. And more than from the matter of indulging the emotional and the sentimental prohibition against sending such an old to prison, I shall not give your disciples and followers the morbid satisfaction of regarding you as a martyr.

I shall not, therefore, adopt the government's suggestion because I think it might be a highly dangerous one. We have far too many cults with their masters and their prophets, their leaders. I know also of the little German who was sentenced to jail and wrote a book there that was instrumental in bathing the world in more blood than has ever occurred since the beginning of civilization. So I will not send you to prison at this time.

I will endeavor to construct the sentence against you and your company without imprisonment but so that it will be designed to effect what is the intention of the verdict of this court, namely, to being to a complete stop the promotion of this so-called science in this country.

At 10 a.m. on January 31, 1947 Dinshah appeared for his sentence. The Spectro-Chrome Institute was fined $1,000 on each of the twelve counts. Dinshah himself was fined $1,000 on each of Counts 1, 2, and 3 and imprisonment of one year on each of those counts, to run consecutively. However, the prison term was suspended and Dinshah was placed on five years of probation. Additionally, he was fined $1,000 each for Counts 4, 5, 6, 7, and 8, and there were several conditions of probation.

Dinshah found the court's reasoning flawed and was personally deeply affronted by its despicable comparison of him to Hitler. Hitler was a murderer, an incarnation of evil who ruthlessly exterminated six million Jewish lives; he, Dinshah, was a caring, incorruptible, devout man who selflessly devoted his life to ameliorating suffering humanity, to saving lives! Dinshah promptly gave an oral notice of appeal. This was followed on April 8, 1948 by a "Petition for Writ of Certiorari to the United States Circuit Court of Appeals for the Third Circuit" submitted to the U.S. Supreme Court. With his Writ

Dinshah hoped to have the higher court review his case as tried in the lower court.

Dinshah wrote that he was handicapped in the trial owing to "the total destruction by fire of all the records and property" of himself and his institute.

Dinshah inferred the prosecutor was condescending. For instance, in his direct examination Dinshah attempted to explain the science behind his healing art to support the statements on the label and the prosecutor said: "Do we have to have all this high school chemistry and physics? Can't we get down to this machine over here?" to which Dinshah replied "That leads to the machine." Dinshah wrote that the objection of the prosecutor about "this high school chemistry and physics was untenable on the face of it, because it was quite possible that some members of the jury might not be familiar with such subjects."

Dinshah wrote that "the law gives an accused a 'jury of his peers,' which in this instance was declared by the Court itself as being too unskilled for the task upon them to adjudge." He asserted that the prevention of experimental demonstrations and "the unskillfulness of the Court, the prosecutor and the jury was an open admission of the miscarriage of justice and a serious violation" of his constitutional and other substantial rights. He stated: "That in considering expert testimony, the jury should bear in mind that honest differences of opinion exist among practitioners of diverse systems of healing and that such opinions tend to be biased."

Another point Dinshah brought up referred to the court's statement that he had "failed to bring any convincing proof of the value of this system of healing except as it came from the lips of 100 or 150 poor souls who ... swore that they felt themselves relieved by the use of the mechanism."

In his argument on this point Dinshah wrote "The true value of any new device may be enunciated reliably by those who used it according to its technique and instructions. Those witnesses who came voluntarily by the scores, day after day, from all over the country, at their own expense and are designated by the court as 'dupes', were the logical ones who spoke about the device from their personal experience, many of them having suffered for years as serious ailments and were declared as hopeless cases by the orthodoxy. They were affiliated Students of the Petitioner Corporation and still stand by their Institute."

Dinshah compared the case to that of Galileo Galilei, "the great astronomer and physicist who was ordered to be tortured for heresy by the Inquisition because of his statement about the motion of the solar system. He was asked to apologize openly, to escape punishment imposed as a sentence by seven cardinals. He did, but, when he rose from his knees he stamped on the ground and exclaimed 'Eppur si muove!' ('Yet it moves!').

Dinshah further argued that :

'Misbranding' at its worst is in the statute a 'misdemeanor' and to inflict upon a researcher, an inventor, a known scientist, a man who lived only to work for the World, by dedicating his life to suffering humanity and whose such services were in demand and were appreciated by a certain group of people, who religiously believed the chemical effects producible on the human body by the color waves of the device was to make the crime a felony, far beyond the scope of the statute. The judge said 'There is evil in this thing.' That opinion created the severe penalty.

The court had also mandated that he dissolve the non-profit Dinshah Spectro-Chrome Institute; turn over all his Spectro-Chrome literature, including all his books on his healing science, to the government for destruction; that he discontinue directly or indirectly dispensing free guidance with respect to his healing system; and that he stop editing the *Spectro-Chrome* publication. Dinshah offered arguments against each of these requirements, and that at all reasonable times he had freely and voluntarily opened his records for inspection to proper authorities of the government. With respect to the order that he cease editing his publication, he pointed out that the order "is a flagrant violation of the First Amendment of the United States Constitution."

In May 1948 the U.S. Solicitor General of the U.S. Department of Justice responded to Dinshah. Following the brief was the statement "The petition for a writ of certiorari should be denied."

With the Solicitor General's response the axe came down on the Spectro-Chrome originator. But he found the brief to be so fallacious that on May 13, 1948 he wrote back to the justices of the U.S. Supreme Court.

"The Respondent presented no argument in support of its Opposition," he wrote, "that would affect the grant of the Writ of Certiorari; instead it made many untruthful and evasive statements."

Altogether, Dinshah's appeal, Writ of Certiorari and response to the brief submitted to the Supreme Court justices in response to his brief show that he was frustrated by how everything had turned out for him. Could it have been prejudice against him? He was essentially waging a war against the powerful medical profession and huge drug industry since his system largely removed the need for doctors and drugs. Can any one person fight these behemoths? Dinshah was a fighter to the end but it didn't make any difference. He was completely shut down. The verdict was sealed and if Dinshah so much as promoted or taught his healing science in any way, he would, if caught, go to prison.

Despite the future of Spectro-Chrome appearing doomed, there would be a bright spot coming up for Dinshah. On August 23, 1947 his wife, Irene Grace, would after having seven sons give birth to her and Dinshah's first daughter. Shireen Dinshah was born at 8:23 a.m. Dinshah was 73 years of age.

27

SUNSET YEARS

Immediately following the expiration of the probation period, Dinshah, at the age of 76, formed the Visible Spectrum Research Institute. Through this vehicle he hoped once again to try to achieve his goal. But the government was determined as ever to prevent him from getting started again.

In a 1957 newsletter to members of the Institute, Dinshah's last such correspondence, he reported the events of October 27 in his research building. FDA agents came to his office to inspect the premises. Then they requested the names and addresses of the members using the color projectors and records of the payments he had received. Dinshah refused to give them the information they wanted. He told them he had an exclusive patent for the color projector granted by the United States Patent Office and requested their superiors to make a full investigation of his science. The officers departed.

Dinshah continued in his newsletter, telling how the next day he was barraged with long-distance telephone calls from members of the Institute complaining that federal officers were coming into their homes and asking all sorts of questions about their relationship with

Dinshah and about Spectro-Chrome. Dinshah apprised them of their legal rights, citing the Bill of Rights of the U.S. Constitution, Article Four. The FDA agents determined who had Spectro-Chrome machines by going to the transportation companies and getting the names and addresses from the bills of lading. One stalwart woman from Illinois told the government agents that she was so satisfied with the results of Spectro-Chrome that she was going to order another projector.

In 1958 the government secured a permanent injunction prohibiting Dinshah from selling his machines and books in interstate commerce. He then confined his distribution to the state of New Jersey. Dinshah pointed out one great omission in the Bill of Rights: "There is no *freedom of healing.*"

At the age of 85 Dinshah said: "I have been persecuted all my life for merely serving suffering mankind but I shall continue to serve as long as there is breath in my body."

Dinshah now lived alone in the Institute building, where he slept in a small bedroom. The only furnishings were a bed, a chair, a bureau, and a small organ which he played daily. His wife lived next door with their children (he wanted this arrangement to spare them the continuous harassment to which he was subjected), and she brought his meal once a day. Dinshah looked lamentable in his appearance and sparse surroundings yet one could always sense his total dedication and single purpose of life — that of helping suffering mankind.

Dinshah never wavered from his convictions and would give his viewpoints at any opportunity. For instance, while eating out once Dinshah requested a vegetarian dinner but given boiled vegetable topped with an egg. He refused it and the hostess was summoned. Dinshah asked her if she menstruated. She replied: "Yes." He then asked her if her husband licked it. Startled, the woman could not speak for a moment. Dinshah continued, "You are eating the menstruation of a chicken when you eat an egg. Eggs produce stinking gases in the body."

On Saturday, April 30, 1966, at the age of 92, Dinshah passed away. His shell was cremated the following Monday in Philadelphia and the ashes were scattered in Malaga Lake.

Dinshah left the worldly domain never having realized his dream of Spectro-Chrome germinating into the ubiquitous panacea for ill health that he boldly envisioned. After decades of fighting forces that vigorously challenged him, he indubitably had to come to terms with the fact that his beloved science would not take hold in his lifetime. Perhaps he took consolation, however, by having read and heeded the words of his hero and acquaintance Nicola Tesla, who in 1934 wrote:

> The scientific man does not aim at an immediate result. He does not expect that his advanced idea will be readily taken up. His work is like that of a planter — for the future.

AFTERWORD

The authors first learned about Dinshah through their father, Philip Rachlin, who attended one of the health practitioner's Spectro-Chrome lectures in the Philadelphia area in the 1950s. Philip had wanted to pursue a career as a physician, but his family was too poor to even send him to college and he abandoned his dream. He eventually became a business owner, but maintained an avid interest in medicine.

At first, Philip thought it was preposterous that shining a colored light on an ailing part of the body could cure it, but over time he became open to the healing method's possibilities, keeping in mind that there was actually a science to the application of colored lights on diseased organs. Over the next several years Philip continued looking into Dinshah's health methods, which included dietary and lifestyle recommendations, and eventually began adhering to these regimens himself with beneficial results.

Growing up, Philip's four sons were amused by their father's clunky light machine and even wondered at times what made him such an avid user of it. Two of his sons became physicians, but never seemed to have much more than a passing interest in this unorthodox form of medicine. Eventually however, Philip's son, Steven, a medical doctor who specializes in alternative medicine, became intrigued by Dinshah's light therapy and began using it on himself privately (never in his practice because Spectro-Chrome therapy is not FDA-approved and is not considered an accepted standard of care). As it turned out, he credits Spectro-Chrome therapy with saving his wife Jeanne's life, as well as his own.

In 1996 Dr. Rachlin's wife, Jeanne, had Stage 2 breast cancer. She had a mastectomy, but was reluctant to undergo chemotherapy and radiation therapy and spoke with Dr. Rachlin's colleague, physician and bestselling diet author Dr. Robert Atkins. As a result of their conversation, she pursued Dinshah's holistic therapy including Spectro-Chrome and his Rational Food of Man diet, and never had a recurrence of cancer; today she is in excellent health.

In January 2005, Steven Rachlin suffered a severe cerebral hemorrhage in the right hemisphere of his brain. So catastrophic was the injury that hospital physicians did not expect him to survive. However, shortly after he was admitted to the hospital, his wife Jeanne brought in his Spectro-Chrome light projector and tonated his head (with indigo) to control the bleeding there and to his heart (with purple) to reduce his blood pressure. Dr. Rachlin not only survived his cerebral hemorrhage but continues to practice medicine today, although he has some paralysis on his left side.

It is easy to see why Dinshah was branded a quack in his lifetime: who would take seriously the notion that colored lights can cure diseases? Yet to some extent conventional medicine already accepts this proposition, and research is continuing today that lends further support to this idea. For example, blue light has long been used to treat jaundice in newborns. A recent study in the scientific journal *Plos One* showed that blue light therapy can also provide long-term control of chronic atopic dermatitis. A recent article in *Harvard Health Publications* posited that seasonal affective disorder could be successfully treated with light therapy. Researchers at Ohio State University recently found that hamsters exposed to red light at night showed less symptoms of depression than when exposed to white light; they felt this could be important to humans who work night shifts and may be subjected to mood disorders. Neuroscientists at MIT recently discovered that by using yellow and blue light they could shut down abnormal brain activity in patients with epilepsy, Parkinson's and traumatic brain disorders. Another recent study in *Plos One* showed that the human body emits visible light at very low intensities at different times during the day (this is exactly what Dinshah said over a hundred years ago and is part of the basis of his science). Numerous additional studies could be cited but the point of all this is that the benefits of light therapy are being discovered more and more today. However, no credit is given to Dinshah nor is there any investigation of his science, either because researchers do not know of him or because there is still a stigma attached to his name and his work.

Despite emerging scientific evidence that lends support for light healing, the authors would like to emphasize that they have no agenda in telling Dinshah's story, and they are, they can assure you, educated and enlightened individuals who do not believe in "miracle cures" or anything of that nature! The authors merely believed they were privy to a little-known and engrossing story (they have a library of his documents and have been learning about Dinshah for decades) and they only wished to write a straightforward but compelling biography.

There is no doubt that some readers will come away from reading the book wondering if in fact there any validity to Dinshah's science. Perhaps now, in the 21st century, medical scientists with open minds might be inclined to do research on Dinshah's healing system.

Billions of dollars are spent annually on research to cure cancer and many other diseases, but not only have no cures been found for many of these diseases, the incident rates for some diseases are increasing. If Spectro-Chrome proved to be an inexpensive natural alternative treatment for diseases it could revolutionize medicine.

Given emerging scientific support for Dinshah's work and society's being more open than ever before to holistic alternative treatments, it seems the time has come for a thorough, fair and impartial investigation of this science.

Dinshah was born in 1873 and has been dead for over half a century now, but his legacy continues today in the form of The Dinshah Health Society, a nonprofit scientific and educational corporation in Malaga, New Jersey, run by his sons, Darius (the president), Roshan, and Jal. As trustees they are not paid, and the Society has no salaried employees. The IRS has recognized it as a nonprofit corporation, and it does not pay taxes or collect sales tax.

Many sites on the Internet today deride Spectro-Chrome and label Dinshah a quack. And yet his legacy is the stellar health results obtained by physicians and other health professionals as well as laypersons all over the U.S. from Spectro-Chrome treatments. With judicial decisions from the 1940s preventing the subsequent practice of Spectro-Chrome and the healing system never being scientifically studied, Dinshah has largely faded in the public memory. Yet with legions of people who were allegedly cured when conventional medicine adjudged their conditions terminal and hopeless, we thought his story was important and deserved to be told.

BIBLIOGRAPHY

Babbitt, Edwin D. *The Principles of Light and Color: The Classic Study of the Healing Power of Color* (edited by Faber Birren). Secaucus, NJ: Citadel Press, 1980.

Bealle, Morris A. *Medical Mussolini*. Washington, D.C.: Columbia Publishing Co., 1939.

Dinshah, Darius. *Let There Be Light* (Ninth Edition). Malaga, NJ: Dinshah Health Society, 2007.

Dinshah Health Society Newsletter. Letter Number 135. June 28, 2017.

Ghadiali, Dinshah P. Colonel. *Dinshah Naturalization Case Clearing Contested Citizenship*. Malaga, NJ: Dinshah Spectro-Chrome Institute, 1944.

Ghadiali, Dinshah P. *Spectro-Chrome Metry Encyclopedia* (Fifth Edition). Malaga, NJ: Dinshah Health Society, 2003.

Ghadiali, Dinshah P. *Triumph of Spector-Chrome* (Second Edition). Malaga, NJ: Dinshah Health Society, 2000.

Ghadiali, Dinshah P. (editor). *History of Spectro-Chrome, Vol. 1*, 1922-1929, Malaga, NJ: Spectro-Chrome Institute.

Ghadiali, Dinshah P. (editor). *History of Spectro-Chrome, Vol. 2, 1930-1935*, Malaga, NJ: Spectro-Chrome Institute.

Ghadiali, Dinshah P. (editor). *History of Spectro-Chrome, Vol. 3, 1936-1938*, Malaga, NJ: Spectro-Chrome Institute.

Ghadiali, Dinshah P. (editor). *History of Spectro-Chrome, Vol. 4, 1939-1941*, Malaga, NJ: Spectro-Chrome Institute.

Ghadiali, Dinshah P. (editor). *History of Spectro-Chrome, Vol. 5, 1942-1944*, Malaga, NJ: Spectro-Chrome Institute.

Ghadiali, Dinshah P. (editor). *History of Spectro-Chrome, Vol. 6, 1945-1947*, Malaga, NJ: Spectro-Chrome Institute.

New York Times (1896) "Says X Rays Are Not New: Views of Dinshar Pestonjee Ghadially, the Indian Scientist, Principle An Old One, He Declares," 11 March, p. 16.

New York Times (1919) "Favors Scant Bathing Raiment for Women," 18 July, p. 11.

Pancoast, S. *Blue and Red Light, or, Light and Its Rays as Medicine Showing That Light IS the Original and Sole Source of Life, as it is the Source of All the Physical and Vital Forces of Nature, and That Light is Nature's Own and Only Remedy for Disease and Explaining How to Apply the Red and Blue Rays in Curing the Sick and Feeble; Together With a Chapter on Light In the Vegetable Kingdom.* Philadelphia: J.M. Stoddart & Co., 1877.

Pleasanton, Augustus James. *The Influence of the Blue Ray of Sunlight and Of the Blue Colour In the Sky In Developing Animal and Vegetable Life: In Arresting Disease and In Restoring Health in Acute and Chronic Disorders to Human and Domestic Animals As Illustrated by the Experiments of Gen. A. J. Pleasanton and Others Between the Years 1861 and 1876.* Philadelphia: Claxton, Remsen & Haffelfinger, 1876.

Spectro-Chrome, Vol. 1, 1922-30, Philadelphia, PA: Spectro-Chrome Institute.

ABOUT THE AUTHORS

Steven M. Rachlin, M.D., is an internist who specializes in complementary and alternative medicine. He made national headlines in November 1994 when he delivered a premature baby on board a TWA flight (#265 from JFK to Orlando) and performed CPR to save the baby's life. For several years he had a weekly radio show on WEVD (1050 AM) in New York City called *Health 2000*, which covered such topics as nutrition and preventive medicine. Dr. Rachlin has lectured widely to both professional and lay audiences over the years. He received a B.A. from Syracuse University and his M.D. degree from the University of Bologna, Italy. He did his medical residency at Winthrop University Hospital in Mineola, New York.

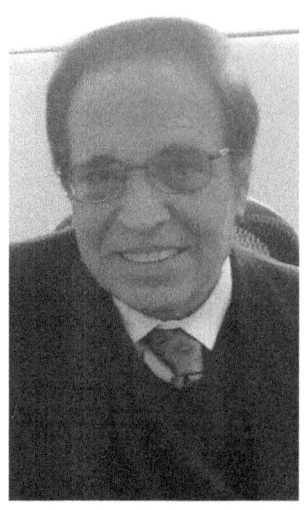

Steven M. Rachlin, M.D.

Harvey Rachlin (brother of Steven Rachlin) is the author of many books, including *The Making of a Cop, The Making of a Detective, Scandals, Vandals, and da Vincis,* and *Lucy's Bones, Sacred Stones, and Einstein's Brain,* which was adapted for the smash-hit History Channel series, *History's Lost and Found.* His first book, *The Songwriter's Handbook,* sold over 50,000 hardcover copies in thirteen printings, and was the best-selling book on the subject for many years; and his *Encyclopedia of the Music Business* won the ASCAP-Deems Taylor Award for excellence in music journalism, was named Outstanding Music Reference Book of the Year by the American Library Association, and was recommended by composer Henry Mancini on the 1984 internationally-televised Grammy Awards. His music books have been praised (on their back covers) by Elton John, Aaron Copland, Johnny Mathis, Pat Boone, and the Academy Award-winning songwriters Burt Bacharach, Sammy Cahn, Marvin Hamlisch, Henry Mancini, Richard Rodgers, and Jule Styne.

Harvey Rachlin has written more than 200 newspaper and magazine articles, with publication credits such as *The Wall Street Journal*, *The Times* (London), *The New York Times*, *The Jerusalem Post*, *The Writer*, *Law and Order*, *Publishers Weekly*, and *Westchester Magazine*. He has appeared on hundreds of radio and television programs and is a lecturer/professor in music business at Manhattanville College in Purchase, New York. More information on his books can be found on his web site: www.harveyrachlin.com

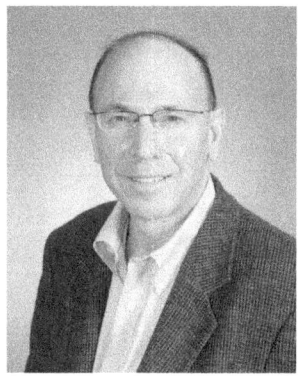

Harvey Rachlin

PICTURES

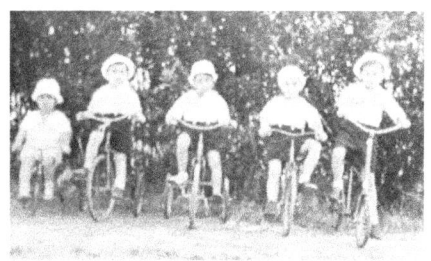

Pictured here on bicycles, circa 1936, are five sons of Dinshah P. Ghadiali and his wife Irene Grace; from left to right (youngest to oldest): Sarosh, Jal, Darius, Roshan, Cyrus. Not pictured is another son, Hom (born in 1934). Two more children would later be born: a son, Noshervan (born 1937), and a daughter, Shireen (born 1947)

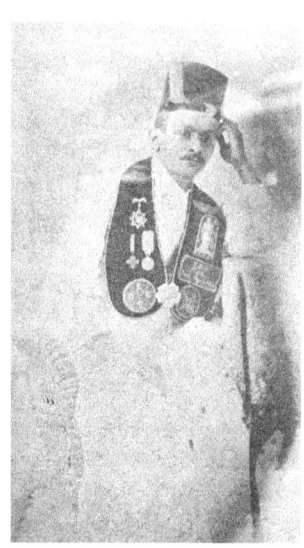

Dinshah P. Ghadiali, about 23 years old, in 1896 when he came to America to lecture on X-rays. An article about him that appeared in the March 11, 1896 edition of The New York Times said he was "known in India as the 'Parsee Edison'".

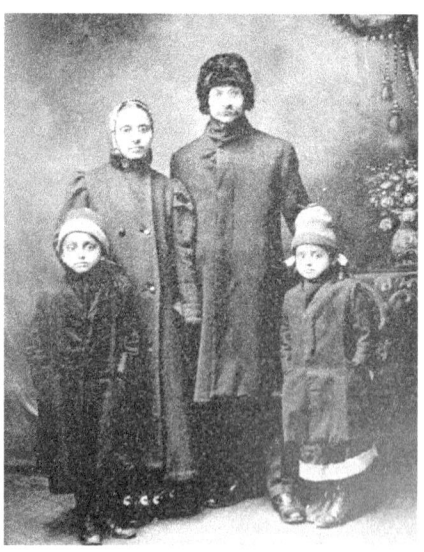

Dinshah and Manek in January 1912 with their two children: Khushcherer and Kashmira.

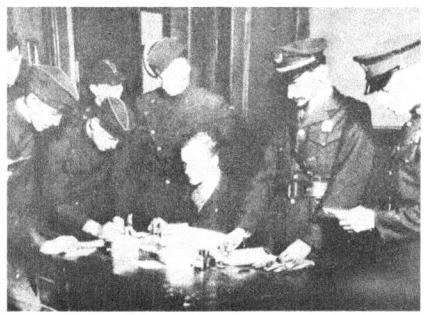

Dinshah P. Ghadiali, standing second right, in 1918. He was Governor of the New York Police Aviation School.

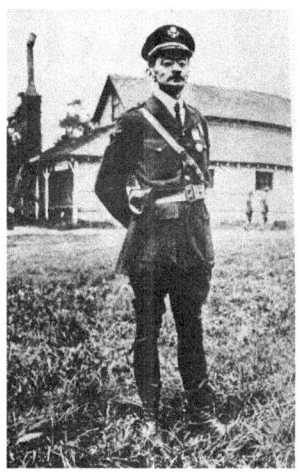

Col. Dinshah P. Ghadiali, circa 1918. He received commissions of colonel and commander of the New York Police Reserve Air Force.

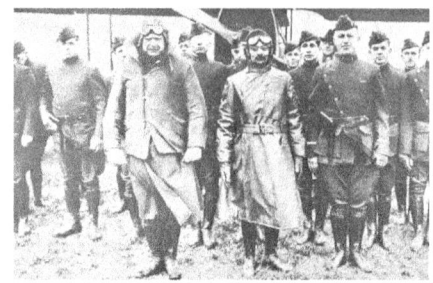

April 26, 1919: Dinshah (front right) on the field at the inauguration of the first air mail delivery of the New York Police Reserve Air Service (New York to Philadelphia) flight.

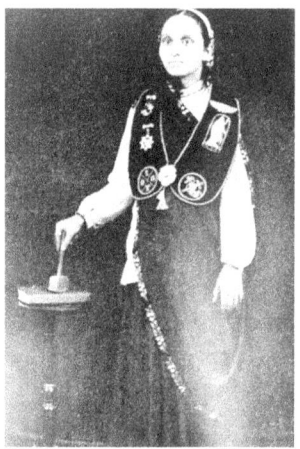

Manek Hormusji Mehta, first wife of Dinshah P. Ghadiali.

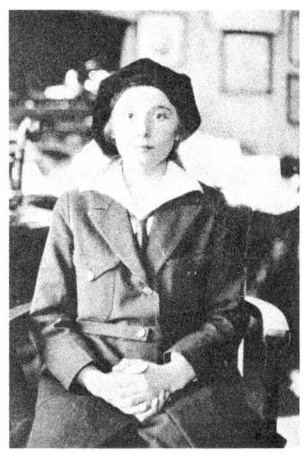

Irene Grace Dinshah, who married Dinshah P. Ghadiali
on March 14, 1923.

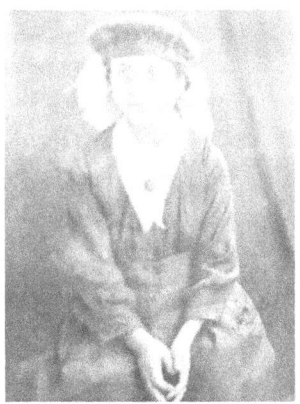

Kashmira Dinshah Ghadiali, Dinshah's beloved
daughter, born in Surat, India in 1904. She was her
father's faithful assistant and a talented poet and
writer.

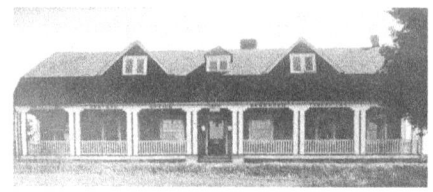

Spectro-Chrome Institute (main office shown) in Malaga, New Jersey as it was when the 23-acre property was purchased by Dinshah in 1924.

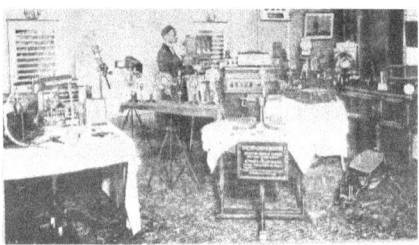

Spectro-Chrome class demonstration set-up, circa 1925.

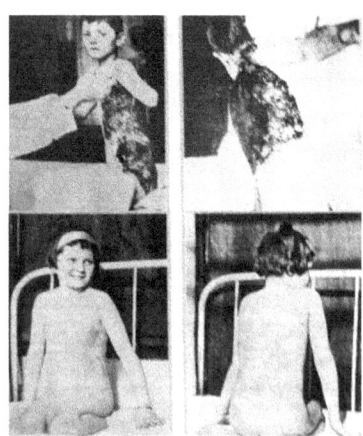

Top: Grace Shirlow, 8 years old, two weeks after she was admitted to Philadelphia Woman's Hospital in December 1923 with severe burns over most of her body. Below: Grace Shirlow, about 18 months after she was tonated by Dr. Kate Baldwin, Chief Surgeon of Philadelphia Woman's Hospital. The young burn victim was released from Woman's Hospital around May 1925.

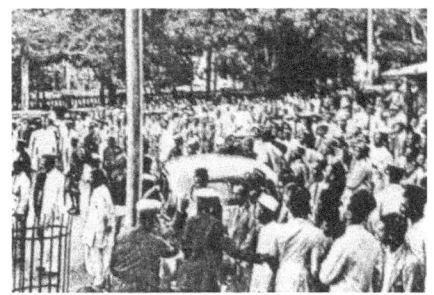

In 1939 Dinshah presented several lectures in India where he spoke on prohibition. Unruly mobs were often against his views.

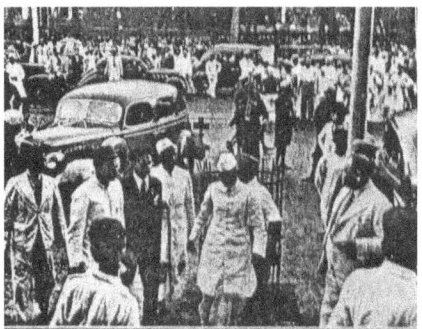

A crowd watches Home Minister of Bombay State Kanaiyalal Maneklal Munshi and Dinshah P. Ghadiali (dressed in black) arriving at a lecture.

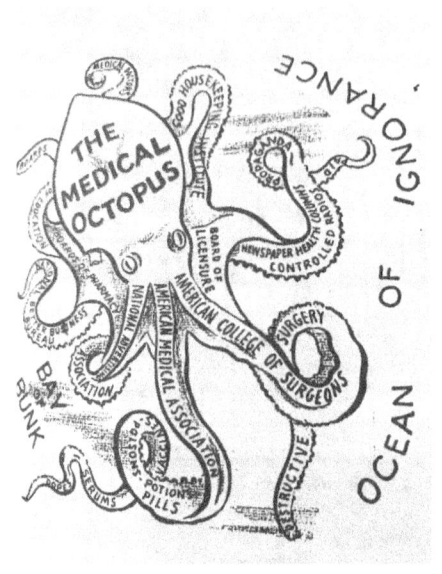

A cartoon illustrating Dinshah's view on medical
control in the U.S.

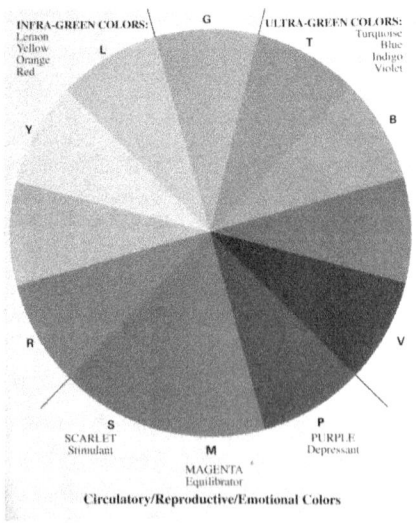

Color wheel

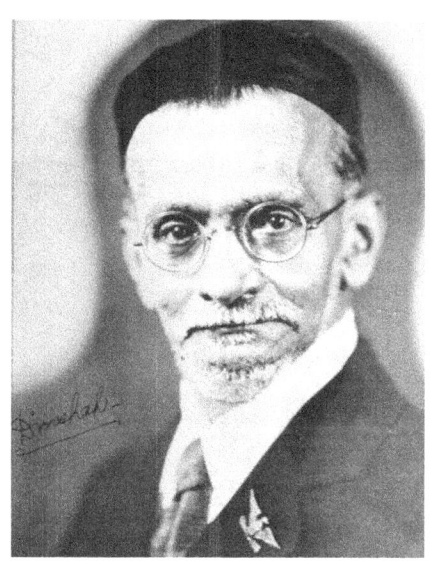

Dinshah Pestanjee Ghadiali, 1873-1966.

ACKNOWLEDGMENTS

This book is the result of many years of steadfast labor and searching for a publisher who would be willing to take on the controversial subject of color-light healing. But just as the times have changed from the days when the U.S. government tried to prevent Dinshah from becoming an American citizen because he was deemed not to be Caucasian, so too, do we hope that the scientific community in these more broad-minded times will be open to investigating color-light healing for any potential health benefits.

Our list of acknowledgments is relatively short, but we hope that in turn each acknowledgment carries great weight.

Our foremost appreciation goes to the Dinshah Health Society for its generous support.

The authors are also indebted to Liesbeth Heenk and Amsterdam

Publishers for bringing our manuscript to publication. Liesbeth is an extraordinary publisher and was always a great pleasure to work with; she gave our book a home and our gratitude to her cannot be overstated. We hope that her belief in us and our book is validated by any scientific breakthroughs this book may inspire.

Steven Rachlin would like to express his love and gratitude to his wife Jeanne and daughters Stephanie, Aimee and Amanda; son-in-law Greg Munves and grandchildren Ben and Bradley. All were supportive throughout the arduous process of writing this book. He is also grateful to Vianne Lamendola, who has been his devoted and trustworthy medical assistant for over 25 years.

Harvey Rachlin's son Glenn is a boundless source of joy and inspiration in his life, and he thanks him and his wonderful daughter-in-law Rebecca for their wholehearted support. He is also profoundly grateful to his significant other, Alysa Sasson, who illuminates his world with her own bright shining light, and to her terrific children Danielle and Barry.

Finally, the authors would like to extend their appreciation to those who lived the story of this book, and were maligned or persecuted in one form or another for what they firmly believed was a veritable medical means to help suffering humanity. Whether they were right or wrong remains ultimately to be seen, but surely theirs is a dramatic story which the authors believe needed to be told. The list of people who lived the story is long but includes, primarily, Dinshah and his wife Irene Grace and daughter Kashmira, Dr. Kate Baldwin and Dr. Martha Peebles. For all those we've left out, we offer our apology. While we understand that some might see light-healing as quackery, our goal is only that this book may inspire open-minded investigations of Dinshah's healing therapy.

Finally, on a personal note, our utmost gratitude goes to our mother Mazie Rachlin, and to our father Philip Rachlin for his unswerving belief in Spectro-Chrome and for introducing us to the amazing story behind it. The scientific book is still not out on color-light healing. History awaits.

Title: Color War. Dinshah P. Ghadiali's Battle with the Medical Establishment over his Revolutionary Light-Healing Science

Authors: Steven M. Rachlin, M.D., and Harvey Rachlin

ISBN 13: 9789492371645 (ebook)

ISBN 13: 9789492371638 (paperback)

Publisher: Amsterdam Publishers

Copyright text © 2018 Steven M. Rachlin, M.D., and Harvey Rachlin

Picture Credits Photos by permission of the Dinshah Health Society.

Back cover On the back cover and in the list of pictures is a color wheel that was created by Dinshah Health Society as a modernized version of Dinshah P. Ghadiali's six-pointed star, which listed all the colors in the Spectro-Chrome colored-light healing science but did not show them. The color wheel has the twelve colors of the Spectro-Chrome system: red, orange, yellow, lemon, green, turquoise, blue, indigo, violet, purple, magenta, and scarlet. The wheel is meant to give a visual representation of color opposites: red/violet; orange/indigo; yellow/blue; lemon/turquoise; purple/scarlet. Green and magenta do not have opposites as they are medians, or stabilizing colors.

According to the Spectro-Chrome system, each color in the wheel has certain qualities that correspond to a specific element; every element (as can be seen when analyzed by a spectroscope) gives off characteristic color waves under atomic disintegration, so therefore by tonating (irradiating) the appropriate color on an area with a problem, the disorder (disease) can be normalated, or brought to a state normal for that person.

DISCLAIMER

This book is a biography and is intended only to tell the life story of Dinshah P. Ghadiali. This book is not intended to render medical or health advice, and the authors and publisher assume no responsibility for the application of any information contained in the book.

www.ingramcontent.com/pod-product-compliance
Lightning Source LLC
Chambersburg PA
CBHW071717120626
46550CB00001B/268